Establishing
a Heart Failure
Program

THE ESSENTIAL GUIDE

Establishing a Heart Failure Program

THE ESSENTIAL GUIDE

Michael McIvor, MD

With assistance from Ray and Jeff Howard

THIRD EDITION

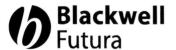
Blackwell Futura

© 2007 Michael McIvor
Published by Blackwell Publishing
Blackwell Futura is an imprint of Blackwell Publishing

Blackwell Publishing, Inc., 350 Main Street, Malden, Massachusetts 02148-5020, USA
Blackwell Publishing Ltd, 9600 Garsington Road, Oxford OX4 2DQ, UK
Blackwell Science Asia Pty Ltd, 550 Swanston Street, Carlton, Victoria 3053, Australia

First published 2007

1   2007

ISBN: 978-1-4051-6750-5

Library of Congress Cataloging-in-Publication Data

McIvor, Michael.
    Establishing a heart failure program: the essential guide / Michael McIvor,
with assistance from Ray and Jeff Howard. – 3rd ed.
        p. ; cm.
    Includes bibliographical references and index.
    ISBN-13: 978-1-4051-6750-5 (alk. paper)
    1. Heart failure clinics.   I. Howard, Ray, 1936- II. Howard, Jeff, 1963- III. Title.
    [DNLM: 1. Heart Diseases–therapy.   2. Health Facilities–organization & administration.
3. Practice Management–organization & administration.   4. Program Development.
WG 166 M478e 2007]
RC685.C53M39 2007
362.196′120068–dc22

                                                                        2007010317

A catalogue record for this title is available from the British Library

Commissioning Editor: Gina Almond
Development Editor: Fiona Pattison
Editorial Assistant: Victoria Pitman
Production Controller: Debbie Wyer

Set in 10/13 Palatino by Aptara Inc., New Delhi, India
Printed and bound in Singapore by Fabulous Printers Pte Ltd

For further information on Blackwell Publishing, visit our website:
www.blackwellcardiology.com

The publisher's policy is to use permanent paper from mills that operate a sustainable forestry
policy, and which has been manufactured from pulp processed using acid-free and elementary
chlorine-free practices. Furthermore, the publisher ensures that the text paper and cover board
used have met acceptable environmental accreditation standards.

Contents

Acknowledgments

Creating a book is a big task. Even though this text stands on the shoulders of the two editions of my previous works on this topic, much of the text had to be rewritten and updated to reflect current thinking in this rapidly changing field. My own efforts were supported by the work of a number of others who were critical in bringing this book to reality. I thank Ray and Jeff Howard who reviewed and edited Chapters 5 and 6 on the financial projections for a heart failure program. Their expertise in this area reassured me that I wasn't leading readers astray in the sometimes confusing world of reimbursement for medical services. Although any errors in the text are my sole responsibility, I thank Susan Neill and Denise Fuller for reviewing my work and pointing out areas of the book that could use improvement. Their insights as experts in delivering heart failure care guided the content revisions from my previous books in this therapeutic area. Likewise, thanks are due to Karen Sommers for preparing the manuscript and to Marcello Benedicto for preparing the figures. I also would be remiss if I didn't thank Gina Almond at Blackwell for having enough confidence in me to lead the effort of championing the book to her organization, and Fiona Pattison, also at Blackwell, who turned my manuscript into a book. I think that we can all be proud of the book that represents the fruit of our collective efforts.

Introduction

Like most physicians, I have been taking care of patients with heart failure (HF) beginning when I was in medical school, continuing through my cardiology fellowship at Johns Hopkins Hospital, and then in private practice. Like other diseases such as HIV disease or cancers, HF is a chronic, lethal, incurable disease. But unlike those other conditions, most medical physicians feel comfortable caring for HF patients unassisted. We all are familiar with the basic precepts of the treatment of HF: therapeutic lifestyle changes, the basic pharmacologic therapies that prolong the life of HF patients, and the newer strategy of life prolonging device therapy. However, every critical examination of HF therapy in the United States has documented that we are not using all the weapons in our arsenal. We know what works, yet we are not systematically applying these proven therapies.

The issue, I think, is the relentlessly dynamic pace of chronic HF. The continual, frequent adjustments in HF therapy are not the strength of physician-delivered therapy. Physicians have the training to rescue the acutely ill patient in the intensive care unit with pulmonary edema. After the acute phase of the illness passes, frequent one-on-one physician visits are simply too expensive to be the standard of care. While there is evidence that when subspecialists provide the HF care, outcomes are improved, most HF care in this country is provided by primary care physicians whose resources are stretched thin. As a result, HF remains the number one reason for hospitalization in the Medicare population. Despite significant advances in our therapeutic options, from the data we have there has been little significant impact in the mortality of HF patients since the 1950s [1].

We now know that there is a better way to treat HF. Formal HF programs for outpatients have consistently resulted in fewer hospitalizations, and in some studies, lower mortality for HF patients. At UCLA, after physicians were told that they were being assessed for the frequency with which they discharged HF patients on angiotensin-converting enzyme (ACE) inhibitors, ACE inhibitor use increased to 73%, at a time when the national average was below 50%. However, when a disease management program was applied to these same patients using nurse case managers, ACE inhibitor therapy on discharge increased to 96% and was sustained for 6 months. The disease management approach in this study resulted in an 83% reduction in HF hospitalizations during those 6 months. The therapy used was simply standard therapy; the difference was the systematic application of this therapy [2]. The experience of my first HF disease management program duplicated the UCLA experience, reducing annual HF hospitalizations by 71%.

My involvement in this therapeutic arena began obliquely. In the mid-1990s, it became clear to me that my patients who were participating in HF research trials were receiving a higher level of care than those who were not in such trials. I was not consciously treating these two groups differently, but in the research trials, aggressive care is mandated by protocol, and the nurse research coordinators were seeing these patients more frequently than with usual care. In one HF trial in which we participated, patients were seen weekly for the first 14 weeks of the protocol. Under such circumstances, it is difficult for an HF patient to "fall through the cracks." I was impressed that even patients in the placebo group had very few hospitalizations or even exacerbations of their symptoms. It was clear to me that the clinical improvement of these patients with advanced HF was that the research nurses had essentially created an HF disease management program, and it worked. My experience is not unique. Recently Dr Barry Levine told me that his HF program at the San Francisco VA also resulted from the efforts of his research coordinators doing HF research trials.

After deciding to start a formal HF program in 1995, based on my experiences with research patients, I found little guidance on where to start assembling the nuts and bolts to build a disease management program. As a result, that first program was a matter of on-the-job training, with resultant bumps and bruises being suffered until I had the experience necessary to discern the best way to manage an HF practice. To share my experiences, I wrote *Blueprint for Heart Failure: A Physician's Guide to Establishing a Heart Failure Center in the Private Practice Setting*. The response to the two editions of the book convinced me that I had discovered a real educational need. Subsequently, I developed and chaired a 5-year program of hundreds of day-long Blueprint for Heart Failure CME symposia around the country, teaching thousands of healthcare professionals how to effectively care for patients with chronic HF in today's healthcare environment. It has been a real education and privilege on my part to work with HF programs of all sizes and in all stages of development. While the disease remains the same, the strategies applied to HF care reflect the intelligence and creativity of talented members of the medical community.

This book updates my previous books both from my own ongoing experiences in treating patients with HF and what I have learned from others through the Blueprint program. I hope it allows you to avoid the mistakes I've made (freeing you to make totally new mistakes of your own as you develop your own program!). As always, I appreciate feedback, questions, and hearing of your own success stories. I can be reached at 900 Central Avenue, St Petersburg, Florida, 33705.

References

1. Levy D, Kenchaiah S, Larson MG, *et al*. Long-term trends in the incidence of and survival with heart failure. *New Engl J Med* 2002;**347**:1397–1402.
2. Fonarow GC, Stevenson LW, Walden JA, *et al*. Impact of a comprehensive heart failure management program on hospital readmission and functional status of patients with advanced heart failure. *J Am Coll Cardiol* 1997;**30**:725–732

Companion website

Be sure to visit the companion website for this book to download the following forms for use in your own heart failure center

www.blackwellpublishing.com/McIvor

Minnesota Living With Heart Failure Questionnaire

The Kansas City Cardiomyopathy Questionnaire

Berlin Questionnaire

Epworth Sleepiness Scale

Sexual Health Inventory for Men Questionnaire

Nutritional Assessment Form

Dietary Recall Diary

Food Frequency Checklist

Protocol ACE Inhibitors

Angiotensin Receptor Blockers

Hydralazine/nitrate protocol

Aldosterone Antagonists

β Blockers

Telephone Management Guidelines

Telephonic Patient Encounter Algorithm

CHAPTER 1

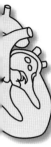

Is a heart failure program the right choice?

Your practice or hospital has been treating heart failure (HF) patients as long as you have been in existence. We now know some of the limitations of how we have treated HF in the past, and more effective ways to approach this disease have been identified. However, before proceeding with the effort and investment of setting up a new way of doing things, you will want to be sure that a formal HF program is right for your patients, your practice, and your community.

Is a heart failure program right for your patients?

Heart failure (HF) remains a challenging condition to treat. In fact, it is sometimes even a difficult condition to define. Nonetheless, HF remains a cardiac epidemic, afflicting 5 million Americans, with 500,000 new patients joining this cohort each year. It has taken some time for us to accept that HF is not the episodic disease that it at first seems. It is in fact a chronic, progressive disease punctuated by episodes of decompensation. While our initial clinical focus was on stabilizing a patient's hemodynamics during these decompensations, it has become clear that many therapies that reduce HF symptoms do not impact long-term prognosis. The pillars of HF therapy are now aimed at improving survival rather than simple symptom relief. Getting a patient on a regimen of evidence-based doses of the neurohormonal antagonists, though, is not easy. One is always fighting hypotension, hyperkalemia, the cardiorenal syndrome, and so on. The titration of the medical regimen does not end when target doses are achieved. As in many chronic diseases, patient management is characterized by ongoing up- and down-titrations as the clinical picture changes. It is difficult for a physician working alone to maintain the schedule of very frequent visits needed by the patient with advanced HF.

Getting a heart failure patient on a regimen of evidence-based doses of therapy is not easy

In addition, the value of patient self-care in HF is well established. In the brief encounters that patients have with physicians during an office visit, teaching a patient about sodium budgets, fluid budgets, and self-management of diuretics is very challenging, if not virtually impossible.

In our program we say that the new math of HF is that $7 \times 1 = 0$, and $3 \times 3 = 2$. In other words, if we teach seven things to a patient once, he or she is likely to retain nothing. If, on the other hand, if we teach three things three times, we can expect most patients to remember two of them. Unfortunately, in the current healthcare environment, the pressure on physician time necessitates that this time be spent on activities that require the training and experience of a physician. Patient education is not one of those activities that can only be performed by a physician. Therefore it will always be a lower priority (than say, a cardiac catheterization or a transesophageal echocardiogram, which do require a physician), no matter how important education is to patient outcomes.

The use of heart failure programs has now risen to the level of national guidelines

The practical choice with which we are left is to provide incomplete care or to leverage physician resources by using nonphysicians. The latter is preferable, and the emergence of formal HF programs to meet this need is no longer new or unproven. In fact, the use of HF programs to deliver care has now risen to the level of national guidelines. The 2005 American College of Cardiology/American Heart Association guidelines give the highest level of recommendation to treating HF patients with formal HF programs [1]:

> Multidisciplinary disease-management programs for patients at high risk for hospital admission or clinical deterioration are recommended to facilitate the implementation of practice guidelines, to attack different barriers to behavioral change, and to reduce the risk of subsequent hospitalization for HF.

The 2006 Heart Failure Society of America guidelines likewise support the use of HF programs [2]:

> Patients recently hospitalized for HF and other patients at high risk should be considered for referral to a comprehensive HF disease management program that delivers individualized care....

The acceptance of the superiority of this new model of care represents an international paradigm shift. The 2005 update to the European Society of Cardiology HF guidelines also addresses not just the therapy to use in HF, but how to deliver that care [3]:

> An organized system of specialist heart failure care improves symptoms and reduces hospitalizations and mortality of patients with heart failure.

While there is general agreement, then, that the preponderance of evidence supports the widespread adoption of HF programs, there are a number of specific approaches that have been put forward, none of which has proven to be the superior method of managing HF patients. Low-tech and high-tech telemanagement systems, hospital nurse case managers, home health HF nurses, and dedicated HF clinics have all met with varying degrees of success. In this book I will present my experience with my own programs and with others I have seen be successful. Other types of programs may also be effective, but I know firsthand that the methods presented here can improve patient outcomes.

Is a heart failure program right for you?

It is one thing to know the strengths and weaknesses of various approaches to HF care. It is quite another to know which approach will work for you. The premise of this book is that the most cost-effective and clinically effective way to treat chronic HF in adults is a formal HF disease management program. In spite of my personal enthusiasm for the disease management strategy, after talking with physicians across the country, I have learned that this approach will not work for everyone. You may be accustomed to being the sole caregiver for patients under your charge. The shift to managing an HF team that provides this care is a big step philosophically and emotionally. The skill set required is different than what I acquired in medical school and requires spending a considerable amount of your professional time being a program builder, a teacher, and an administrator. The physician still drives a disease management program. However, in the model I propose here, there are on average four patient contacts with non-physicians for every physician contact. In traditional models of care, all the responsibility ultimately rested on the doctors' shoulders. That is still true, but in the disease management model, much of the decision making is done, and much of the care is delivered, by nonphysicians. This makes some physicians very uncomfortable.

In the disease management model, there are four patient contacts with nonphysicians for every physician contact.

A reasonable analogy here is the military. While the admiral carries ultimate responsibility, and it is his or her decision to move the fleet from point A to point B, the admiral doesn't physically steer the ship. Everyone knows the chiefs run the navy. The first "go/no go" decision in considering the establishment of your HF program, then, is to know yourself and your style of patient care. If you must be both the admiral and the chief, if you can only be comfortable if you control all aspects of a patient's care, it is unlikely that you will be happy providing that care in the setting of a disease management program. There may be (and are) randomized clinical trials demonstrating the benefits of HF programs. These trials mean nothing, though, if the model doesn't work for you. I personally find that I function more effectively when supported by an HF team of nonphysicians. I recall trying to run an HF practice in one hospital totally on my own. It quickly became apparent that I couldn't use aldosterone antagonists such as spironolactone in that setting. Being swamped with all of the details of HF care, I was certain that I would be unsuccessful in monitoring potassium levels as frequently and diligently as prudence would dictate. I felt it was just a matter of time before a patient developed an avoidable episode of serious hyperkalemia. The Canadian experience with spironolactone bears out my concern. After the RALES trial established the benefit of spironolactone in HF, prescriptions for spironolactone in that country quintupled. Unfortunately, hospitalizations for hyperkalemia tripled, with deaths from hyperkalemia also increasing threefold [4]. I was sure that my experience would be the same. However, over time the program grew, and could support additional staff. Once I had HF nurses helping me, I developed an aldosterone antagonist treatment protocol for initiating and following patients on this therapy. Within months, I was comfortable placing patients on aldosterone antagonists, referring the patient to the appropriate HF nurse, and not giving the issue another thought. I am comfortable with the fact that when treating chronic disease, the chiefs run the navy. In fact, under my direction, the chiefs do a superior job running the navy.

Physicians who run all care through their own hands, by definition, limit the number of patients they can see and how often they can see them.

Acute illness is a different situation. As an interventional cardiologist, I know it has been extremely gratifying for me, when presented with an ill patient suffering from an acute coronary syndrome, to be able to draw on my training as a physician to assess the patient's problem, determine a course of action with clear therapeutic goals, and then to achieve those goals. With patients who are acutely ill, the physician personally provides the critical steps in patient care—in this case revascularizing the threatened myocardium. With chronic disease states, the situation requires a different clinical solution.

Physicians who insist that all care run through their own two hands, by definition, limit the number of patients that they can see and how often they can see them. They become, as we discuss later, the "growth-limiting resource." An HF disease management program should be customized to address the growth-limiting resource of a particular program. Physician time, expense, and availability are common growth-limiting resources. The HF care team leverages that scarce and expensive resource, essentially allowing the physician to concentrate on activities that truly require the training and experience of a physician, and to virtually be in many places at once. This is a critical function of the HF program. However, not being personally involved in every clinical decision represents a significant loss of control and the acceptance of a degree of uncertainty. If you are a physician who is uncomfortable relinquishing clinical decision making to other members of your team, you will likely not be successful in building an HF practice based on the disease management model. Likewise, if training staff to assume roles as physician extenders is not your strength, your program may struggle.

Without doubt, a critical piece of a successful HF program is the physician medical director. While much of this book will focus on the impact of the nonphysician component of the HF team, an HF program is much more likely to be successful if it is led by an enthusiastic and visionary medical director. There are many leadership roles in HF programs that are best accomplished by a physician. These include not only setting the program's medical style of HF care, but also overcoming the political and logistical challenges that all new programs face. In the absence of a physician committed to the task, I have found that it is difficult to establish a sustainable program, and as a result much time, effort, and money is wasted. Taking on this responsibility can be a difficult choice for the busy clinician. Beyond that, the medical director must be convinced that an HF program is the right solution for the local circumstances in which the program will exist. An important part of that decision is whether the medical director has the temperament for running such an endeavor. Physician, know thyself. If a disease management program is not a good fit for you, there are other solutions to delivering HF care. If, on the other hand, this model of care appeals to you, this book should be of help.

Is a heart failure program right for your community?

Each medical community is a little different. You are in the best position to know how a new HF program will be accepted. A cardiologist or hospital depending on referrals as a source of patients for the program needs to assess how the referring physicians will feel about physician extenders delivering so much of the day-to-day care. I must say that this was something of an issue when I started my first HF program. The situation today is more accepting than it was even a decade ago, but even today this is something that should figure into your decision whether to begin an HF program. Further, whether establishing a program within a physician practice or a hospital, there are likely to be other stakeholders. A series of questions naturally arise. Considering the situation of a physician practice:

Will other partners turn over their HF patients to the program?
What will be the impact of the program on workflow in the office?
How long will the practice need to support the fledgling program until it is financially viable?
How much of a distraction will setting up the program be (training the staff, developing protocols, etc.)?

The local conditions will determine the sort of HF program that best suits your community. Resources are always finite and will determine whether you develop a comprehensive program or a "boutique" program that only meets specific needs, such as education or drug titration. Limitations on the time that the medical director can spend on this effort, or on the size of the physical facility, or fiscal restraints all determine the scope of your program. The question then becomes not just if an HF program is right for your community, but what type of program is aligned with the goals of your practice or hospital. Focusing initial efforts on the most pressing needs of the community (rather than duplicating services already available) and being realistic about what can be achieved have helped me be successful in my programs, whether in a private practice or hospital setting.

You are in the best position to know how a new HF program will be accepted in your community.

Once your program is established, patients appreciate the more intense education, evaluation, and follow-up they receive. Typically, patients become attached to the HF staff who spend so much time applying the $3 \times 3 = 2$ principle discussed above. Patients with advanced HF rightfully see their cardiac condition as a predominant health problem. The presence of HF has implications for many of a patient's comorbidities (e.g., the selection of β-blocker or angiotensin receptor blocker, the use of nonsteroidal anti-inflammatory agents). Ultimately, the expertise patients perceive in your staff on such issues will make your patients the best ambassadors for your program, and community acceptance and appreciation of your efforts will follow. The most successful HF programs I have seen are prudent enough to never take the community for granted, working hard to keep referral sources, patients, and the community at large "in the loop."

Summary

HF therapy is difficult and complex, and is best provided by many hands working in unison. The clinical efficacy of HF disease management is now accepted, and the approach has been incorporated into US and European HF guidelines. This is an effective delivery system of HF care for patients. That does not mean that an HF program will be universally accepted and successful. The decision to proceed with establishing such a program will be based on matching the particular features of a specific HF program to the temperament of the physician leading the effort, as well as the specific needs for HF care of the local patient and medical community.

References

1 ACC/AHA 2005 Guideline Update for the Diagnosis and Management of Chronic Heart Failure in the Adult. *J Am Coll Cardiol* 2005;**46**:1116–1143.

2 Adams KF, Lindenfeld J, Arnold JMO, *et al*. HFSA 2006 Comprehensive Heart Failure Practice Guideline. *J Card Fail* 2006;**12**:10–38.

3 Swedberg K, Cleland J, Dargie H, *et al*. Guidelines for the diagnosis and treatment of chronic heart failure: full text (update 2005). *Eur Heart J* 2005;**26**(11):1115–1140.

4 Juurlink DN, Mamdani MM, Lee DS, *et al*. Rates of hyperkalemia after publication of the randomized aldactone evaluation study. *New Engl J Med* 2004;**351**:543–551.

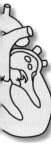

CHAPTER 2

A formula for the success of your heart failure program

Even once you decide a formal heart failure (HF) program is right for you, your patients, and your community, success is not assured. To be successful, your HF program needs enough patient flow to justify the investment of human and physical capital, a physician champion to provide leadership and vision, a staff with the enthusiasm and skill to bring that vision to reality, a thoughtful approach to program design, and a clear definition of what it means for your program to be deemed successful.

At this point I will assume that you have decided that proceeding with the development of an HF program is the right thing for you, your patients, and your community. The next step is to devise a strategy that maximizes your chances of developing a sustainable program. Over the last several years, I have had the opportunity to meet with thousands of healthcare professionals who are involved in HF disease management programs at various stages of development. Some of these programs have been successful; others have not. Success was not assured solely by a commitment to the notion that the disease management program was the best way to care for patients. Success or failure easily depended as much on the organization and infrastructure of the program. Commitment and the right formula are both required. So what are the essential components of a successful HF program?

Keys to a successful HF program

- An HF patient cohort of sufficient size
- An enthusiastic and visionary physician champion
- An independent and professionally competent full-time staff
- A model of care that leverages your unique growth-limiting resources
- An early selection and commitment to program benchmarks

Key component one: an available population of heart failure patients

The model that I will describe in this book is a volume-driven model. It can be successful in both the fee for service and capitated payor environments.

However, if you have only 12 HF patients in your practice, it is unlikely that the time and effort of setting up an HF program will be rewarded. The first key to success in any payor environment is a patient flow that justifies the staff necessary to provide the resource intensive care that HF patients need. One would think that this should not be a problem in light of the fact that HF is the leading cause of hospitalization in the Medicare patient cohort. It is the prevalence of HF that has put this disease on the radar screen of payors and hospitals. Nonetheless, many programs fail because of a lack of patient access. I have seen a surprising number of HF programs that are struggling because there are only a handful of patients in the program.

HF care is resource intensive; for an HF program to be sustainable, there must be sufficient patient flow to support those resources.

There are often political or logistical obstacles that limit patient referrals to an HF program. This can be true for all programs, but is a particularly important issue for hospital-based HF programs. I have encountered many hospital programs that have a few dozen indigent patients as their entire patient cohort. This is not a viable scenario. On the other hand, why should physicians send their HF patients to a hospital-based program and forego the revenue associated with caring for these patients?

There are strategies to apply to this problem. In my opinion, the medical director setting up the program must find the program's "growth-limiting resource." (GLR) If, as in this case, the GLR is patient access, addressing that problem should be the major focus of the program. First, the experience of working with the program must be easy for referral sources. The procedure of making a referral must not only be effortless, but it must also be a pleasant and rewarding experience for referral sources. I was recently visiting a new HF program at a hospital in the Midwest. There was a committed physician in place as medical director. A nurse practitioner had been brought on board as clinical director of the program. During my visit, a primary care physician approached the clinical director with a referral of an inpatient about to be discharged. She told the referring physician that she had reviewed the chart, and there was no recent echo or BNP. Further, from what she could tell, the patient wasn't sick enough to be referred to the program. This was not an example of how to win over referral sources to the program.

The successful HF program must have the capacity to see new patients, today if need be or, at the very least, in the next day or two. The program should exude not only competence in HF care, but also enthusiasm to become the community leader in this therapeutic area. The HF program experience must be a win for the patient, a win for the referring physician, a win for the hospital, and a win for the HF program itself to be successful over the long-term.

Even a hospital program that welcomes new referrals with open arms can struggle with the issue of patient access. Again, why should anyone refer an HF patient to a hospital HF program and forego the revenue of caring for the patient's HF? No physician thinks that he or she is doing a substandard job in HF care. How can the HF program do a better job? One hospital that had encountered this problem told me of their innovative solution. The hospital had started an HF program headed by a nurse practitioner and had been surprised that the cardiologists in the four groups on staff weren't referring patients.

The hospital decided to lease the nurse practitioner running the HF clinic to the various cardiology groups. Group A leased the nurse practitioner on Mondays, group B leased her services on Tuesdays, group C on Wednesdays, group D on Thursdays, and a group of internists on Fridays. Each group could now refer their patients on their given day, have them treated by protocols devised by each group, and bill for the services of their leased employee. With this strategy, the perceived loss of control of patient care and loss of revenue were removed in one fell swoop. Not surprisingly, the program became a success, once there was a win–win situation for patients, physicians, and the hospital. The hospital was wise enough to realize that a key to success was patient access and addressed this GLR.

Key component two: the physician champion

The HF programs that I have seen fail most often do so due to the absence of a visionary and enthusiastic physician champion. Typically, the failed program consists of a cardiology practice or a hospital turning to a physician extender, such as a nurse practitioner or physician assistant, and telling that person to "start a heart failure clinic." Without a physician champion to provide a consistent and unified vision of where the program is headed, without a champion to make critical decisions in the early phases of the program development, it is unlikely that the program will ever be able to overcome the hurdles facing it in its formation stages. It is likely that only a physician has the political capital to overcome the obstacles all new programs face. Change always generates resistance; the standard bearer that will change minds is usually the physician champion. The importance of a dedicated physician champion cannot be overstated.

In a private practice, the physician champion alone can nurture the program in its nascent stages, protecting the program from the push back that inevitably comes from other (non-HF) staff within the practice, other partners within the practice, referring physicians, area hospitals, and the lay community. The staff of the HF program needs to focus on developing its style of treatment, and then implementing procedures and protocols. It cannot be distracted by the other political concerns of establishing a new business entity. That is the task of the physician champion.

Once the program comes into its own, the role of the physician champion shifts. Now he or she must promote and broadcast the successes of the program to that same staff, those same partners, those referring physicians, the hospitals, and lay community. This may take the form of speaking engagements, participation in the various hospital committees in the community dealing with HF, interacting with patient organizations such as Mended Hearts, or taking a leadership role in professional organizations such as the local chapter of the American Heart Association. The goal is to make your program both the provider of choice and the source of information about HF care.

The physician champion is key. The physician champion alone can nurture the program in its nascent stages, and later must promote the successes of the program to the community.

The physician champion is key. That being said, much of the success of disease management programs involves "getting the doctor out of the loop" of day-to-day operations and letting physician extenders provide the intense education and compliance monitoring, necessary for successful outcomes. However, this does not mean banishing the physician to Siberia. The physician champion is still critical in establishing strategic therapeutic goals for each and every patient, and in providing credibility to the program by assuring that the healthcare product being delivered by the program is of high quality. The physician champion is the shepherd of his or her HF flock. It has been the rare program in my experience that has been successful without these functions being fulfilled by an enthusiastic physician with a special interest in HF.

Medicine needs pioneers, those truly insightful thinkers and believers who create new therapies, often by challenging medical dogma. For example, everyone in the medical community knew that placing a catheter into a beating heart would be a lethal event. We were wrong. Forsman the pioneer was right, and now the cardiac catheterization laboratory is a central element in the evaluation and treatment of heart disease. Everyone knew β-blockers were essentially malpractice in HF. We were wrong. The pioneering Scandinavians were right, and now β-blockers are a pillar of HF therapy.

Medicine needs pioneers to push back the frontiers of our knowledge and to challenge our existing paradigms. Most pioneers fail and most new trails lead to dead ends. It has been very difficult to develop new inotropes that prolong life in HF. The early promise of ventricular reduction therapy for HF does not seem to represent a durable benefit. Still, without pioneers, we would never discover those new pathways that do lead to effective HF therapy.

As the HF expert in your medical community, you do not need to be a pioneer, blazing new trails in HF therapy. You should, however, be a trail guide for your community, reading and interpreting the available data to decide which paths of HF therapy are most promising. This is especially true of controversial new therapies, but HF trail guides also need to continually reexamine new uses for conventional treatments. The change in conventional thinking in recent years about angiotensin-converting enzyme (ACE) inhibitors, β-blockers, and inotropes reminds us to be trail guides with open minds.

It is prudent for the physician champion of an HF program to think of the program as operating on multiple levels. The program must meet the needs of its patients, of course, delivering a solid portfolio of clinical services. The program should also serve as a focal point within a practice or a hospital, establishing the local standard of care.

With each disease management program I have developed in any therapeutic area, there have been partners who did not refer patients. Nonetheless, once my first lipid program was established, the use of combination therapy and advanced lipid testing increased throughout the practice. After building an HF program, even patients not referred to the program were more likely to be on β-blockers and on an optimal dose of β-blockers. Hallway consults on how to use ACE inhibitors in patients with mild to moderate renal insufficiency became common. Early adoption of aldosterone antagonists was practiced widely. The successful disease management program has impact outside its own borders.

The physician champion who projects a nonthreatening image of his or her center of excellence may be surprised to subsequently receive referrals from other competing cardiologists, especially for the complex HF patient who requires advanced therapies. As the local HF expert, the medical community will look to the physician champion for leadership, either overtly or indirectly. A program can be well designed and well staffed with competent healthcare providers and yet still fail if it is not seen by the community as the provider of choice for HF services. This means more than success-fully competing with other providers of HF care. It also means cooperating with those competitors and demonstrating true leadership.

Do the keys of the program need to rest in one pair of hands? One, per-haps two medical directors are the most that an HF program, especially a new program, can accommodate.

It is the role of the physician champion to set such a tone. Acting at such a community level is difficult for some physician champions. This inclusive style may be counterintuitive in a community of competitors and an environment of shrinking medical reimbursement. However, programs that shirked this role of trail guide (typically a monopolistic large group or hospital) have achieved only temporary success. The financial model proposed in a later chapter is a volume-driven model. Some programs rely only on internal referrals. The most successful, however, also draw from external sources of HF patients. Only a trusted trail guide will garner such external referrals.

If your program is truly embracing HF care, it will likely remain several steps ahead of the competition, offering newer therapies, providing better service, and achieving better clinical outcomes at a lower cost for payors. If this is so, there is no risk to being a trail guide. Your program will never get all of the HF patients in your community. HF is such a common disease that is so underdiagnosed and undertreated that there is plenty of work to go around for everyone. I never expect other cardiologists in town to refer NYHA Class I or II HF patients to me. It is a real compliment to the programs that I have established to get referrals of NYHA Class IIIB and IV patients from hundreds of miles away, who need the advanced services we provide. I believe that this reflects on our recognition as enthusiastic community HF trail guides.

Do the keys of the program need to rest in one pair of hands? I have encountered many, many hospital programs that fear offending members of their medical staff and as a result rotate the medical directorship. This is usually an error. It is unlikely that each member of the rotation will have the true interest, temperament, and skill set to take on this role. Further, a rotating or committee approach to leadership rarely provides a unified approach to HF care for the nonphysician staff to follow. In my experience, one, perhaps two medical directors are the most that an HF program, especially a new program, can accommodate.

If there is a committee of 10 cardiologists directing an HF program, no doubt there are 13 opinions on what color the walls should be painted. This is not to say that there shouldn't be widespread participation in setting up and managing the program. It is certainly reasonable to have an advisory committee comprising the various political entities of the medical staff for program oversight. I would emphasize again, though, that the medical directorship should rest in one pair, or at most two pairs, of hands.

Key component three: an independent and professionally competent staff

While a physician champion is the first key step on which to build your HF program, the program will not truly be successful until the staff carrying out most of the day-to-day patient care activities also embraces HF care. Again, the programs I have seen that have been less than successful typically staff the HF clinic with the same physician extender who runs the Coumadin clinic, the lipid clinic, and does the precath histories and physicals. HF therapy is complex and requires considerable energy to successfully implement. A staff that is distracted with other non-HF related duties cannot provide a high-quality HF product.

Most of the staff with whom I have worked have told me when they were hired that they were quite familiar with HF therapy. After about a year or so, invariably they have come back and told me that they never realized how much they didn't know about HF when they started. One cannot know what one doesn't know. While I have used part-time staff in my programs, I believe that the key personnel must have all of their time dedicated to HF care for the program to be successful. There is a lot for the staff to learn, and outside a formal HF program, there are few places for them to learn it. The typical patient in an HF program is ill enough that hospitalization can be justified at each outpatient visit. Finding staff who can be comfortable with such a sick patient population requires the personality of a home health or hospice nurse. Finding staff who are comfortable with aggressive therapies in this patient cohort requires the personality of the critical care nurse. Finding both personalities in the same person is a rare find indeed.

The brain of an HF program is the physician champion. The heart of the program, though, is its staff.

Your HF staff must be both intelligent and independent. Patients who are treated through an HF program achieve success partly through their interactions with the physician, but also through their more frequent interactions with the HF staff in the office and on the telephone. A staff distracted with significant other duties cannot do as good a job with telemanagement.

The staff must exude competence and dependability, especially for patients with more advanced stages of HF.

Training the HF staff takes time. I knew that my first HF program was going to be successful only when the staff began to bring novel ideas to me about providing better care, such as our ACE inhibitor of choice, effective substitutes for NSAIDs, etc.

The bottom line is that both a committed physician champion and a committed staff are necessary for program success. The physician champion is the brain of the HF program. The staff is the heart.

Key component four: a model of care that leverages your growth-limiting resource

Every HF program has a GLR. In physician practices, the most common GLR is the availability and expense of the physician champion. If all the care flows through one pair of hands, you simply cannot see 5000 patients a year. This, however, is not the only GLR that an HF program can face. It could be physical space—you can't see 5000 patients a year in a closet. In a hospital situation, the GLR might be patient flow. If a patient has to register on the first floor, then go to the fifth floor for an ECG, then to the second floor to have a BNP drawn, and finally to the third floor to be seen in a closet, you again can't see 5000 patients a year. The convoluted patient flow in such a program becomes the GLR.

We have already discussed the situation of a hospital HF program that faced the GLR of patient access. The hospital removed the significant obstacle that referring physicians faced of loss of revenue by leasing the nurse practitioner running the hospital clinic to the various cardiology groups on staff. Other approaches to the GLR of patient access would be for an HF program to offer services not offered by anyone else in the community, such as intensive education or advanced therapies.

Every program has a growth-limiting resource. Once it is identified, leveraging that resource is an important key to program success.

Once the GLR is identified, a model of care should be selected that leverages this GLR. Again, in the private practice environment, a common GLR is physician availability. The solution here is to add physician extenders to the care plan. Once leveraged, while a physician sees a patient in one exam room, his or her nurse practitioner can see a work-in patient in the next exam room, a nurse can see a patient in a third exam room for an ACE inhibitor titration visit, an echo tech can perform an echo in another room, and a physician assistant can stand by an exercise test in the next. This approach easily leverages the one pair of physician hands into multiple pairs of hands.

The success of a disease management program lies in part in increasing the number of contact points between patients and their healthcare providers. Frequent contact allows more time for patient education, so patients can begin to manage their own disease. Frequent contact provides opportunities to monitor patients' progress to make sure that they have understood and are successfully implementing therapeutic lifestyle changes and complying with their medical regimens. Frequent contact also maximizes the likelihood that your team will catch early signs of decompensation before these symptoms precipitate a hospitalization. A physician is unlikely to provide these frequent contacts. An HF team will.

Key component five: a commitment to benchmarks

Few HF programs emerge fully formed at the outset, providing flawless care. The program will change as it learns to emphasize its strengths and to improve on its weaknesses. Time after time, though, I have encountered programs that can't decide what they do well and what needs to change. Even if the staff has an intuitive feeling that the program is doing well, it can be very difficult to prove to others that success has been achieved. It is a real shame when a hardworking HF staff cannot prove its worth to partners, to hospitals, and to payors that it does a good job.

If you are not sure how to judge the success of your program, neither will others. At the outset, you are in the best position to define how to measure your success.

Part of the formula for success, then, is an early commitment to a set of benchmarks by which you want your program to be judged. These benchmarks may change as the program matures. For example, in the beginning you might record the percentage of your patients on evidence-based therapy, or the degree to which your program adheres to national HF guidelines. As your program grows and months go by, you might measure echocardiogram parameters, serial B natriuretic peptide measurements, 6-minute-walk distances, or quality-of-life questionnaires. As time goes on, you might add the frequency of HF hospitalizations. Often, separate benchmark patient visits are needed to collect this data.

I am convinced that successful HF programs regularly measure benchmarks and use this data to help prove to the world that the investment of resources in the program is a good investment. During my *Blueprint for Heart Failure tutorials*, a common need raised by established programs was help measuring outcomes. Unfortunately, in the rush to get started, this issue is often overlooked initially, and programs are later unable to justify their existence over time.

Summary

While each HF program has unique features that address the specific needs of their community, there are common features of the successful programs that I have encountered. A sustainable HF program will need a large enough cohort of HF patients, an enthusiastic and visionary physician champion, an independent and intellectually curious staff that embraces HF care, a model of care that addresses the growth-limiting resource (GLR) facing the program, and an early commitment to collecting data on the parameters by which the program wants to be judged. Later in this text, I will discuss the need to incorporate this formula for success into a flexible business plan. This plan will articulate the goals of the individual HF program, and lay out the pathway the physician champion intends to use to achieve these goals.

Taking the first steps toward building your heart failure program

CHAPTER 3

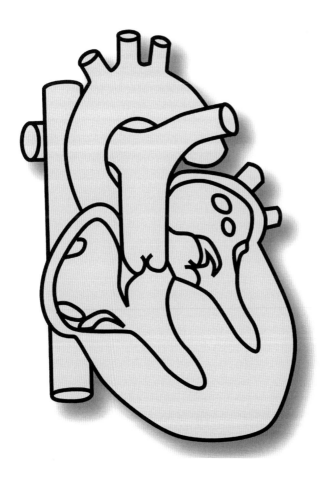

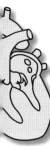

First steps: a business plan for your heart failure program

Building a successful heart failure (HF) program entails an investment of considerable time and effort. It only makes sense to carefully plan out your strategy for success. Putting your ideas to paper in a business plan can help clarify your thinking and avert costly errors.

So, you think that an HF disease management program is an attractive proposition. The next step is to put your ideas to paper. This is a surprisingly difficult step. While you may have a clear image of the program you envision for your practice or hospital, laying out your master plan in a way that makes the benefits of the program obvious to all readers is a challenge for most of us. The devil is in the details, as they say.

I'm convinced that your HF program's chances of success are better if you and your key team members share a common vision about what your program is trying to accomplish. A business plan will help you decide what your program will try to accomplish, or rather what it will be, as well as what it will not be. Many programs that fail are plagued by disagreements about program goals. These disagreements can dissipate program resources in the critical start-up phases of operation. A business plan gets you and your staff on the same track, and then lets you know if you are still on track as your program grows.

Many of my partners in the past have felt that this step is unnecessary, but I have found that writing a business plan is a very valuable activity. In addition to HF programs, I have started coronary heart disease prevention programs, clinical research programs, and medical education programs. The business plan I wrote at the outset of each of these endeavors focused my thinking and focused my presentations to my partners on the need for and goals of the new program.

A business plan will help you decide what your program . . . will be, as well as what it will not be.

Just as you would do for a new business you might propose to venture capitalists, your plan should explain to your partners why they should invest in an HF disease management program rather than, say, buying another nuclear camera or opening a new branch office for the practice in a growing suburb. Unlike the funding request for venture capitalists, though, your HF program proposal seeks to enhance the core business of your practice or hospital, rather than create a new business with an exit strategy for the investors (e.g., being acquired by others or becoming a publicly owned company). That is your advantage.

Your practice partners have invested in the practice. The business plan should reflect that your HF program is a well thought out idea that will enhance the return on their investment. Much of the plan, though, is written for you and your HF staff, rather than your partners. Your plan, if well written, should be a living document, a template helping you to make critical decisions about both foreseen and unforeseen issues and opportunities as your program matures.

Many HF programs that I have seen have gone awry because of unforeseen opportunities that were financially and professionally attractive, yet were not consistent with the initial goals of the program. Pursuing these opportunities can spread the resources of a new HF program too thin to sustain the core mission. A well thought out business plan is a living document that will serve as a touchstone to help you evaluate such new opportunities.

Contents of your business plan

- Executive summary
- Mission statement
- Guiding principles of your program
- History of HF care in your practice
- The HF marketplace in your community
- Organizational structure of your program
- Financial pro forma
- Five-year projections
- Opportunities and threats
- Summary

The mission statement

The first step in creating a business plan is to form a mission statement. I would suggest that you spend some time thinking about your mission statement. Some corporations take 6 months or even a year to compose this statement of purpose. Most physicians I know don't see any value in crafting a mission statement; in fact, many view the whole idea as a waste of precious business planning time. I disagree. Your mission statement distills what you envision your program will become. An effective mission statement should tell you and your staff who you are and who you are not; where you are and where you want to be. Let's look at the utility of some types of mission statements.

Mission statement

It is the mission of XYZ HF program to address the needs of HF patients within the XYZ practice.

This is the sort of mission statement I see most physicians write. I agree that whatever time was invested in coming up with such a mission statement may not have been warranted. It is not the least bit helpful. It gives very little direction. What is the scope of the program? What needs are to be met? All needs? How much staff would that take and what would they do? The only guidance I see in such a mission statement is that the patients for the HF program are to come from within the practice. The program, then, should not spend time recruiting patients from outside the practice. The implication is that referrals will come from your partners.

The weakness of this mission statement is that it provides no guidance for how you are going to "address the needs of heart failure patients." This could be anything from telemanagement only, to advanced therapies, to home health nursing. I wouldn't be able to use this mission statement to tell if I am off track later.

A mission statement is often overlooked or, if written, is often filled with platitudes. Such mission statements are not helpful. I have found that I can use a well-written mission statement to help my staff and me to refocus ourselves and keep ourselves on track.

Let's see if we can do better.

Mission statement

It is the mission of XYZ HF program to address the special needs of adult HF patients and their families. Our goal is to prolong life and improve the quality of life of our patients.

With the mission statement as now stated, my staff would know that we focus on the treatment of adult patients. The first HF program I set up was situated within a cardiology practice that was closely affiliated with a pediatric hospital. This mission statement would establish that we did not intend to treat HF in the pediatric population. It also states that as a program we acknowledge that quality-of-life needs may eventually outweigh the need to extend life in HF. Thus, therapies that reduce symptoms but do not extend life would at least be considered in our program. In fact, therapies that reduce symptoms but adversely affect survival might even be considered. This mission statement is an improvement, but I think we can do even better if we want the mission statement to be a true blueprint.

Mission statement

XYZ HF program was established to meet the special needs of adult patients and families who suffer from HF. Heart failure is a chronic, incurable, fatal disease, but we can impact the course of that disease in our patients.

It is our mission to:
• Educate patients and families about the etiology, natural history, and treatment of HF
• Increase the length of our patients' lives whenever possible
• Increase the quality of life of our HF patients through a program of nutrition, medicine, exercise, and advanced therapies, especially when length of life is not the primary objective
• Incorporate our patients into the development of their care plan and to respect their wishes as to what care they receive
• Provide advanced HF care, including new therapies not generally available or used in the medical community, or to secure that care elsewhere if it is not available in our community
• Pursue research initiatives to advance the knowledge base and care of patients with HF
• Develop a tradition of excellence locally, regionally, and nationally for HF care

---

This mission statement is obviously more complex. It is detailed in its guidance of the program. This mission statement commits the program to pursuing state-of-the-art care. It would be just as reasonable to not provide state-of-the-art care, but rather to provide excellent care that meets or exceeds the standard of the community. State-of-the-art care is expensive and resource intensive. There are other more cost-effective alternatives to being state of the art.

For example, your program may be referral based, and in such a model, you might not follow patients over the long-term. Instead, you might make some initial therapeutic changes, outline suggested goals for a patient's care, and then turn care over to home health nurses or primary care referring physicians, especially if the patient comes to you from a distance. In such circumstances, in which the scope of your program does not include long-term follow-up or comprehensive care, it would be harder to commit to providing state-of-the-art care.

Whatever goals you can reasonably achieve are acceptable for your HF program. The mission statement you craft tells as much about what your program is not as it does about what your program is. In my first HF program, we wanted to set the standard for HF care for our community. Beginning with the mission statement, we committed ourselves to a tradition of excellence beyond our community. Being active in regional and national organizations, therefore, would be appropriate. This mission statement encourages our active participation in the American Heart Association, American College of Cardiology, and the Heart Failure Society of America. We also decided to seek to improve HF care for our patients by engaging in clinical research. This commitment was clearly stated in this mission statement.

Your mission statement should be specific and free of platitudes.

In my opinion, your mission statement should be specific and free of platitudes. It does not need to be as long and involved as the third example here, but it should help guide your HF program development and be a benchmark as to whether or not you are achieving your goals. Your business plan should not be seen as commandments carved in stone. It should be a living document, guiding your program's development, but being amended as your program matures and develops its own character and style, confronting unforeseen obstacles and evaluating unforeseen opportunities. Nonetheless, the more your mission statement tells of your program's goals, the more useful it can be to you and your staff over time.

Guiding principles

If a mission statement lays out the strategy of your program, then guiding principles lay out the tactics. The guiding principles in your business plan define how you will reach the goals of your mission statement. For example, let's say that you are setting up your program within a private practice. Your program most likely is not funded by a charitable grant, so you must create a financially sustainable program. Though professionally you want to build an HF center of excellence, you need to do so while being fiscally responsible. Saying so in the guiding principles makes this statement strongly to your staff and will get everyone off on the right foot.

Guiding principles

• XYZ HF program will create and manage a portfolio of programs in education, research, and disease management in HF patients.

• The program will embrace change to continually improve the services it provides to patients of the practice. Our HF program will be a learning organization.

• The clinical disease management program will seek to define the state of the art for HF care in our medical community. We will educate our patients and our colleagues about HF and its treatment.

• XYZ program will have a goal of establishing a regional, statewide, and national reputation for excellence. We will seek to achieve and maintain a position of leadership in the medical community.

• The services of our program will represent high value for our patients and customers as well as high quality. The strategy to increase value will be to leverage physician resources. This will include the use of new strategies, such as nurse case managers, telemanagement, Internet solutions, and intensive protocol-driven therapy in the outpatient setting.

• Our HF program will use a disease management model of prevention, early diagnosis, and early intervention, rather than episodic care.

• Our program will follow clinical outcomes to document our success and to uncover the path to continual program improvement.

• XYZ HF program will be run in a fiscally responsible way. Much of the value of some HF services will be intangible. The aim, though, is not to simply create a self-sustaining program, but to make the program into a profit center for the practice.

• The XYZ HF program will be run in an ethically responsible manner.

• We will treat our colleagues, our staff, and our patients with dignity.

Another guiding principle might state whether you want your program to grow from internal resources only or whether you expect to share your program with partners outside of your group, such as a payor or a local hospital. Such partnerships may be necessary to secure the resources that will enable an ambitious HF program to establish and maintain itself. You will also want to clarify how you will structure and operate the program, e.g., a disease management model in this case. Again, guiding principles are the tactics you will use to achieve the strategies you set out in your mission statement.

Now that the overall strategy for achieving the goals of the HF program you envision have been laid out in the mission statement and guiding principles of your business plan, fleshing out your argument as to how you came to this vision, this strategy, and these tactics is the next step.

The history of HF care in your practice

Your business plan should describe the current state of HF care in your practice and your community. Your partners or your hospital no doubt have been providing HF care to patients since they have been treating patients. Reviewing both the strengths and weaknesses of your practice performance in HF care should begin to make the argument for the development of a formal HF program. If not, this should give you pause. If you are not advancing HF care to the next level with your program, you should probably rethink the project. If your practice is already doing just fine with HF, using your current model of care, why change it? Usually, a practice survey will reveal that the use of ACE (angiotensin-converting enzyme) inhibitors and β-blockers is much lower than your partners or your hospital would predict and desire. Usually, the practice review reveals areas where a formal HF program can do a better job. If not, you might do well to invest your limited practice resources in another venture.

In any case, the review will be useful in validating what has been done successfully for your HF patients and what areas need improvement. A prudent HF program will focus, at least initially, on those gaps of care you can identify that your program can fill. It also makes sense to acknowledge the successes your group has enjoyed in the past.

The HF marketplace in your community

Along with a review of HF care in your own practice or hospital, a market survey of HF services in your area will be important in shaping the scope of your program. Have your dietician call area hospitals to see what services are available (and for what charge). Have your nurses research the area hospital policies on advanced HF therapies, and whether the hospital case managers have already begun working on HF as a priority item to prevent rehospitalizations. There is little reason to simply replicate services already available in your community. A niche for your program may become self-evident after your market survey as you identify gaps in the HF care of your community.

Actually, I have been surprised at how these activities have shaped my programs. The practice review gives credit to your partners where credit is due for good clinical care, and then explains how the group could do better. There may have been practice or hospital initiatives that occurred before you joined the practice. You would be remiss not to review, analyze, and learn from these prior efforts.

A practice review … gives credit where credit is due … and then explains how the group could do better.

Market surveys can sometimes be surprising in that you may be unaware of what is going on HF care in your own community. This knowledge may allow you to avoid wasteful and costly repetition of services. If your program is to be "better," first you have to answer the question, "better than what?" I have started a number of HF programs, and with each market survey, the focus of what I wanted that particular program to become has been sharpened. I was amazed in creating my first HF program to discover what was available in the community. Despite practicing as a cardiologist in the community for 7 years, I had an incomplete picture of the resources available in the community for HF patients until I did a market survey. I would have never predicted this. Shouldn't these programs have been marketing their services to me?

At any rate, the market survey likely will provide a valuable insight on the HF landscape in your community. The information hopefully will bolster your argument as to why your practice or hospital should embrace your HF initiative rather than invest your limited resources elsewhere.

The organizational structure of your HF program

Your business plan should detail your proposed organizational structure. Unlike a business plan for venture capitalists interested in a start-up business, you will most likely not be bringing in a seasoned professional management team to run your HF program. However, you do need to show how you will organize and run this part of your business and what critical HF staff you will need to start. How you intend to use each part of the staff to deliver HF care and what the management structure of your program will be are both important.

This part of the business plan will present the model of care you have selected (and why you picked it), the staff qualifications and training needed, and the physical facility required to provide the services you want to include in your program. The division of responsibility and accountability needs to be clear. I will discuss some possibilities in the following chapters, but each situation is unique, so your plan will address your particular circumstances.

An HF disease management program simply will not work without the right staff.

I have already emphasized that the physician champion of your HF program is a critical component for success. I would be remiss, though, if I created the impression that your HF staff was any less important. An HF disease management program simply will not work without the right staff. The critical members of that staff must be independent self-starters who embrace HF care and quickly bring new and innovative ideas to the physician champion. How you organize that staff will have a great impact on the success of your program.

You may need to begin with part-time staff when the program is too small to be profitable. However, your plan should include milestones that mark when the time is right to make your HF staff full-time and when new staff will need to be added. In the last chapter, part of the formula for a successful program was an early commitment to those parameters by which you want to be judged. The program milestones included in your business plan should be viewed the same way.

In subsequent chapters I will discuss how successful HF programs that I have seen have organized themselves. Your organization, though, will depend on the local environment in which your HF program will exist.

Financial pro forma and 5-year projections

The financial section of your business plan should provide a clear statement of both the realistic costs and conservative projections of revenues. You can use part of the approach from the financial chapters of this book, but you also need to put in the specifics of the costs particular to your situation. What is the salary overhead? Is 90 ft^2/chair in the infusion suite really necessary? What are the data management costs? How will the costs grow over the next 5 years? What are the "go/no go" decision points, and how will decisions on program growth or program cancellation be made? How will success be measured clinically and financially?

A rigorous pro forma will serve as a blueprint for your program. In my programs, each year I have assembled an annual report to update the partners or hospital on how things are progressing. I have used the financial pro forma section of my original business plan when writing these subsequent HF program annual reports as a check on whether the program was on track financially. It is gratifying to be ahead of schedule. Falling behind should be cause for reexamination of your operation.

Others ... will likely read only the executive summary and financial projections of your business plan.

Remember, your practice partners or the stakeholders in your hospital program will likely read only the executive summary and the financial projections of your business plan. The financial analysis needs to be solid and needs to make a strong case for establishing an HF program by showing a clear and credible path to profitability. In this section, you need to address what could go wrong with the program, and the financial milestones presented need to be realistic and achievable. You would like to take a UPOD (under promise, over deliver) strategy for this part of the business plan. An overly rosy scenario could well come back to haunt you if the program stumbles in the early going.

In this spirit, 5-year projections might be a stretch. While in the past I have even seen 10-year projections, some physicians today will point out that in the current healthcare environment, the future is so uncertain that even 5- or even 3-year projections are a challenge. Your plan will reflect your best guess of how you expect your program to perform as far into the future you can clearly see.

Opportunities and threats

Finally, there is the section that lists the strengths, weaknesses, opportunities, and threats of your proposal. What is the upside and downside of investing resources in an HF program rather than another part of the practice? Is now the time? Is the idea of starting an HF program now in your community premature? On the other hand, if you wait, will your hospital lose momentum and the leadership position? Are you ahead of your competitors or catching up? Is the community ready to support this idea? How will this program affect relationships with patients, referring physicians, hospitals, and payors? If you do not proceed, will someone else grab the opportunity? Like the executive summary, here is where you state the case as clearly as you can for your program. If you are unconvincing, maybe you should rethink your strategy or decide not to build an HF program.

Summary

At the very least, with a business plan in hand, your HF program should no longer be a half-baked, poorly thought out idea. Your plan should be a recipe for success. If you take the writing of this business plan seriously, you will probably change your vision of your HF program while you are composing the plan. As you learn more about HF therapy and how programs are being implemented around the country, your thinking will become more focused. As you critically examine the delivery of HF services in your community, your business opportunities should become more apparent. Refining your vision is a good thing and enhances your odds of building an HF program of which you, your staff, and your partners can be proud, and which everyone can support.

Your business plan should be a living document. It should lay out all the aspects of your program that you can anticipate: your goals, your strategy and tactics for achieving those goals, and your expectations for the first several years of your program. A good business plan helps you know where to start, but also guides decision making as your program faces unexpected challenges and helps you know if you are meeting or surpassing the milestones you set out at the beginning.

There is also the issue of the unexpected opportunities your program will no doubt face as it matures. A well-conceived business plan can help you decide how to evaluate these new possibilities. If the new opportunity is in keeping with your mission, you can embrace it. If it is inconsistent with your program's mission, you need to either change your mission or reject the opportunity. A new idea can be good, but if it is outside the scope of what you are trying to do, it can interfere with your core activities, distract the staff, and deplete valuable resources.

Simply put, while a business plan does take time and energy to assemble, a well-conceived plan will payoff handsomely in focusing your efforts later. Many of the HF programs that I have seen fail struggled because the key players of the program were on different pages from the beginning. This is an easily avoidable mistake.

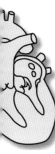

CHAPTER 4

First steps: choosing your model of care

Heart failure care can be successfully provided in a number of ways. The model of care that works best for you will depend on the operating environment of your program, the makeup and experience of your team, the scope of services you offer, and the size of your patient population. Equally important will be defining the growth-limiting resource facing your program, so that you can select a model of care that leverages that scarce resource.

Do we need a new model of heart failure care?

In the traditional model of care, a physician obtains a history from a patient, performs a physical examination, obtains subsequent diagnostic testing, makes a diagnosis of the problem, formulates a plan of therapy, and then monitors the patient response. As physician resources become more precious, this model works less well for the patient with HF. We now have some evidence that giving HF patients the right pharmacologic regimen and advice is not enough. The ACC/AHA performance measures for HF care list a number of interventions clinicians should make when discharging an HF patient from the hospital. A recent registry of about 5000 patients showed that adherence to these performance measures did have the desired impact on 90-day rehospitalization and mortality.

To understand this finding better, let us consider the course of a typical HF patient. Patient Jones was recently discharged after an HF hospitalization. Over the next few weeks, he notices that he is gradually accumulating fluid, gaining 2–3 lb a week. There is a mild increase in symptomatology, but nothing dramatic.

One Friday morning, it becomes clear to Mr Jones that his condition has worsened and he probably won't make it through the weekend without a visit to the emergency department (ED). He calls his physician's office and requests a visit. He is worked into a busy Friday afternoon schedule. There are limited resources to bring to bear at the end of the day, but his physician gives him a prescription for metolazone to supplement his loop diuretic.

By Saturday evening Mr Jones' condition deteriorates further, so he seeks help at the local ED. The ED physician and the physician on call do not know Mr Jones, so he is admitted to the hospital early Sunday morning to "tune up" his HF. The hospital has a critical pathway in place for HF patients. The pathway is designed to minimize length of stay. As a result, before he has made rounds Monday morning (perhaps even before he knows that Mr Jones was admitted over the weekend), the nurses are calling the treating physician to see if Mr Jones can be discharged. Mr Jones is discharged on Monday afternoon with no change in his admission medications. Mr Jones continues his current lifestyle, making the same sodium and fluid indiscretions, and is readmitted 3 months later.

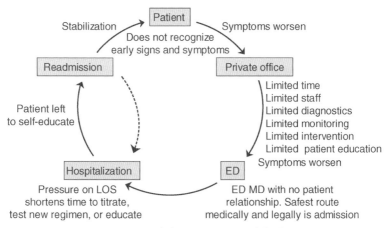

Limitations of the current model of care

The problem here is not a knowledge gap. The treating physician, the ED physician, and the hospital staff all know the key components of HF care. Mr Jones was given the right medications. To break this cycle of hospitalization and rehospitalization, what is needed is education and reeducation followed by intensive monitoring. None of the caregivers in this scenario are tasked with that education and monitoring.

Why is the education and monitoring so crucial in avoiding the ED? The real result of all this work is to empower the patient to recognize the tempo of the HF and to act on changes in his or her condition. The typical HF patient is of Medicare age, so he or she may think their fatigue is the result of advancing age rather than HF. The typical HF patient has an average of three comorbid conditions, so he or she may not be able to tell if their dyspnea is from the chronic obstructive pulmonary disease or HF. An effective HF program will need an education component that teaches patients about the etiology of their symptoms and how to adjust medications based on daily weights and symptoms. Mr Jones ultimately

Traditional model of care

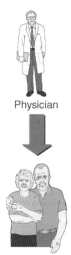

Physician

Patients

will know how to titrate his loop diuretics in response to a weight gain and, better still, he will know how to work within his 2000 mg sodium and 2000 cc daily fluid budgets to stay out of trouble in the first place.

In the traditional model, the physician will teach patients about their HF. I am not saying that we don't. What we usually don't do as well is reeducating and reeducating. We are also less likely to call Mr Jones on a regular basis to check on how he is doing. Patients miss appointments or are lost to follow-up. When doing well, they are seen infrequently and education and monitoring efforts are minimal. The system springs into action only when the patient decompensates, often manifested as a hospitalization. The traditional model is inherently a reactive model rather than a proactive model. There isn't enough time to be proactive with the heavy patient-load of most busy clinicians. The crushing load of existing problems consumes all of the physician's time.

In the traditional model, the physician is a not an HF specialist. This means that the physician is pulled in several directions to meet all the medical needs of her patients, stretching resources thin. By trying to provide all of the HF care herself, the physician limits the number of HF patients that can be under her care. She is the growth-limiting resource. An HF team could share the responsibility of care and see more patients.

The traditional model has been the model of HF care used for decades. It was appropriate when we thought of HF as an episodic disease, and had limited tools to proactively change the natural history of the disease.

As our therapeutic targets in HF now include preventive care, we should consider different models.

The move to systematic care: the physician-driven heart failure clinic

The first move away from the traditional model of care is for a physician to become an HF specialist and develop an HF clinic. The physician leader now commits to devoting a significant portion of his or her professional life to caring for HF patients. In this model, the doctor–patient relationship is still the arena wherein all clinical decisions are made and therapy is delivered. Typically, this is a physician who has taken an interest in HF and so accumulates a cohort of patients in his or her area of interest. This, then, is the physician champion for HF issues for the group practice.

Another example of this model would be an interventional cardiologist who develops skill in stenting carotid arteries. Patients with carotid bruits or TIAs would be referred to this specialist as his reputation grew in the community. Since this procedure can only be delivered by his hands, he is the growth-limiting resource. He would base his decisions upon information he obtained from the patient, the referring physician, or from his review of angiograms, carotid duplex scans, etc. He would apply his specialized knowledge to construct a diagnosis and plan of treatment, and then deliver that care with his own two hands. His office staff might help arrange schedules and give patients pre- and postprocedure teaching, but essentially all the care comes through the physician.

Returning to the case of the HF clinic, the physician who develops a reputation as an HF specialist, adept at balancing conventional as well as new approaches in difficult HF patients, becomes this same type of expert. This specialist devotes a significant portion of time to keep abreast of new developments in HF care, serving as an HF trail guide for the community. Allied healthcare workers could assist the specialist, but all care would flow through the physician. In this model, the physician is still the growth-limiting resource. She can only work so many hours and see so many patients. Her schedule will eventually fill up. Assistants can schedule procedures, call the patients with test results, or run the billing department, but after a point, growth of the program would really depend on adding more HF physicians.

The advantage of moving to this model is that an HF specialist is more likely to systematically use guideline-driven therapy. However, as the practice grows busier, it is unlikely that the physician will continue to spend significant amounts of time on patient education, disease surveillance, or on

Physician-driven HF clinic

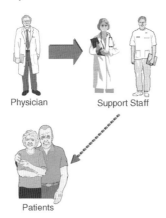

Physician   Support Staff

Patients

preventive measures. These will likely be delegated to the referring physician. In this model, physician resources are so critical to the ongoing activities of the program that these resources must be reserved for what has to be done by a physician, e.g., doing procedures and seeing patients in the office.

Once physician time becomes saturated, this model of care can easily revert to the traditional model of episodic care. With no time for preventive activities, care becomes episode driven; i.e., patients are seen when they are ill. As the program becomes busier, office visits are spaced out over longer periods of time, so that it takes longer to titrate medications to optimal doses, and without regular frequent monitoring, patients are more likely to decompensate.

Having a physician champion to focus attention on HF care is a major step forward from the traditional model. However, except for very small or new HF programs, the physician-driven model is too easily overwhelmed by the needs of sick HF patients. To leverage physician resources, non-physicians must be added to the model.

The physician extender model

An important step toward leveraging physician resources is the physician extender model. An example of this model would be the electrophysiologist with a pacemaker nurse. As in the traditional model, physician resources are best spent doing electrophysiologic studies, implanting devices, and seeing consults in the office or hospital. However, pacemakers and implantable cardioverter defibrillators (ICDs) require an ongoing level of attention after they are implanted. A physician can deliver that care, but it is a time-consuming activity.

A nurse trained in the programming of pacemakers and ICDs can establish and run a clinic for device checks, and can function fairly independently in managing the care of these devices, reprogramming them as needed and monitoring for evidence that a pacemaker or ICD needs to be replaced. The physician can now be in two places at once, doing a consult in one exam room while another patient undergoes a pacemaker check in another room. The pacemaker nurse is a physician extender and allows the program to grow without adding additional physicians. The lower cost of physician extender time allows more patients to be seen and more patient education and preventive services to be delivered.

In an HF program using this model, the physician might see a patient and order carvedilol. The HF nurse could do the appropriate patient education, and then arrange office visits with the nurse for dose titration of the β-blocker. This clearly frees up physician time, as he may only see the patient at the beginning and the end of the drug titration, or if problems arise.

Physician extender model

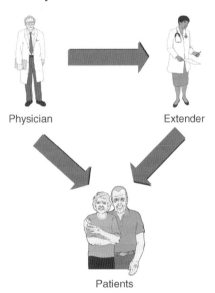

Like the physician-driven HF clinic, in this model the commitment will increase the use of guideline-driven care. In fact, care becomes protocol-driven to assure that it is evidence based. The advantage here, though, is that some of the care is delivered by nonphysicians. In fact, in the drug titration example above, nonphysicians will deliver the majority of the care. In the programs I've seen that are most successful, there are four patient contacts with nonphysician for every physician contact. The physician devises the care and the physician extender delivers the care. As I said in an earlier chapter, the chiefs run the navy, not the admirals. Instead of the physician being the growth-limiting resource, growth of the program is now limited by the number of physician extenders.

The physician extender model is the most cost-effective form of an HF disease management program. It is the model most often selected in the private practice setting, although I have also seen hospitals use it. While this model is effective, it will only work if the physician medical director is comfortable delegating the delivery of HF care to others. Some physicians embrace the concept of the HF team delivering care; others do not. It can be difficult to delegate the task of delivering HF care when the responsibility cannot be delegated. Leveraging physician resources depends on nonphysician participation.

While a physician champion is a key ingredient to a successful program, the champion alone is not enough. A successful HF program will also require a staff of physician extenders to provide the frequent contacts that patients in your program need. Through a program of intense patient education and monitoring, coupled with the aggressive application of conventional and advanced therapies delivered through preestablished protocols, disease management programs provide consistent, cost-effective, high-quality care. Such programs have been shown to deliver superior clinical outcomes

The multidisciplinary team model

In the preceding models, the physician brought specialized knowledge and technical expertise to the healthcare delivery system. In the last few decades, other healthcare professionals began to bring their own specialized knowledge to the table. A dietician, for example, can probably do a better job teaching HF patients about their daily budgets of saturated fat and sodium than I can. A medical social worker is better trained in organizing available resources for a patient to obtain support for prescription medicines, etc. An exercise physiologist has a more detailed knowledge of flexibility training and strength-building exercises for HF patients than a physician is likely to have. An experienced and well-trained HF team can do a superior job delivering HF care.

It is not surprising that the concept of a multidisciplinary team evolved, with the physicians as team captains, but with unique and valuable contributions of each team member being recognized. This approach has worked well in the hospital setting, with the whole team available to meet the patients' needs. Rehabilitation of stroke patients, for example, may use specialists from occupational therapy, physical therapy, speech pathology, dietary sciences, etc. HF patients have multidisciplinary needs as well, and hospitals may already have the necessary assets in place.

Since one physician can be the captain of many teams, physician resources are leveraged even more effectively in this model. Program growth does not depend on adding more physicians, just more teams. Like the physician extenders model, physicians are used in this model for what they do best—bringing their specialized knowledge and technical expertise to bear in directing patient care. Unlike the physician extender model, though, physicians must also develop the leadership skills to harness the talents of the team, not simply to help him do his own work, but to accomplish the objectives of the team in caring for the HF patient.

Multidisciplinary team model

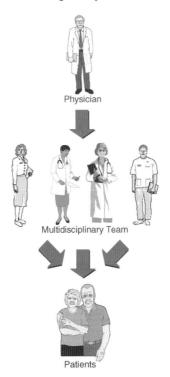

Physician

Multidisciplinary Team

Patients

This, truly, is a new skill. Physicians have always been leaders in healthcare. The interventional cardiologist leads the cath lab team to achieve the goal of successfully delivering an intracoronary stent. In contrast, as leader of the multidisciplinary team, the physician must now assure the quality and efficacy of services she does not personally deliver and might not have the expertise to deliver, such as nutrition counseling and exercise training. The physician must train the team to deliver care by protocols that are in accordance with her conservative or aggressive approach. With multiple caregivers, a consistent strategy or style of HF therapy must still be presented to the patient. This requires training the HF team in a common vision of the goals of HF care, a skill that not every physician has.

As hospitals often have multiple types of healthcare providers on staff, the multidisciplinary team model of care is used in many hospital HF disease management programs. The teams are more available than physicians in the hospital and are less costly than physician time, but teams can still be expensive.

The nurse case manager model

The most successful clinical results reported by HF disease management programs have utilized the nurse case manager model. This is a combination of the physician extender model and the multidisciplinary model. The physician's role in this model is (1) to develop treatment protocols, (2) to perform initial patient evaluations, (3) to establish the goals and plan of care, and then (4) to monitor that care personally and through the HF team. In this model, patients in the program are divided into pods, and each pod is managed by an HF nurse, nurse practitioner, or physician's assistant. The size of the patient pod depends upon the disease severity of the patients and the capacity of the case manager delivering care.

A multidisciplinary team of specialists may be available to the case manager to be utilized selectively as the needs of the patient demand. The case manager "brokers" this care for the patient, rather than having the team decide the care plan. This model is particularly useful when the multidisciplinary specialists are independent contractors with the HF program. If dietician services or cardiac rehabilitation services are outsourced from a hospital, for example, rather than being provided by an employee of the practice's HF program, the case manager model is ideal. Even when the services are all provided internally, the case manager can still help optimize the use of these resources. An NYHA Class I HF patient, for example, may not need physical therapy. On the other hand, an NYHA Class IIIB patient will probably benefit from the services of many members of the team.

The case manager also delivers a substantial amount of care personally to the patient in this model. Most programs find that intensive telephone management (telemanagement) is helpful in achieving improved patient compliance and minimizing hospitalizations. The case manager can

Case manager model

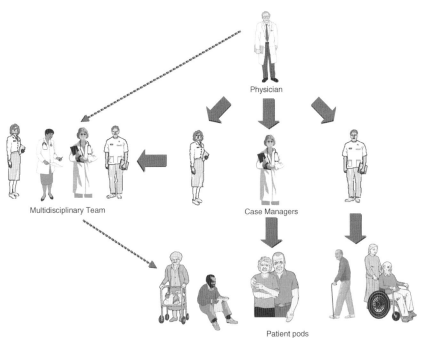

Physician

Multidisciplinary Team

Case Managers

Patient pods

perform this task, or as the patient pod size grows, an assistant can perform the telemanagement and report an increase in signs or symptoms of HF to the manager. Using protocols developed by the physician medical director, the case manager addresses any change detected in patient status according to treatment algorithms. The number of case managers now becomes the growth-limiting resource.

As in the models already described, the case manager will probably see a given HF patient four times for each physician visit. Patient care conferences are used to review patient progress to assure a consistent approach to the HF patient. Major treatment decisions are made by the physician; ongoing titration or adjustment of the therapeutic regimen is done according to protocol.

This model represents a significant departure from the traditional models of healthcare delivery. While the physician–patient relationship is preserved, a significant case manager–patient relationship is also established. When signs or symptoms change, the patient will now tend to contact the case manager. When the physician sees the patient in the HF clinic, it will not be unusual to see that the diuretic, ACE inhibitor, or β-blocker has been adjusted per protocol by the case manager since the last physician visit.

Many physicians are uncomfortable with this loss of control. Every study, though, has shown that physician-directed, case-manager-delivered care produces superior clinical results as measured by patient quality of life, patient compliance with medical regimens, an increased functional capacity, and decreased rates of hospitalization for HF.

Choosing your model of care

There are a number of options I have laid out in this chapter for your program from which you can choose. How do you pick? Very few HF programs are pure forms of these established models of care. Depending on your staffing pattern and the talents of the individuals on your staff, roles will vary in providing HF care to your patients. The "best" model for you will depend on your local circumstances. The first consideration is what you want to achieve with your program. If yours is a hospital program that seeks to reduce hospitalizations in 50 HF patients who are "frequent fliers" consuming excessive healthcare resources, then the traditional model might work for you. Physician time will not be the growth-limiting resource for 50 patients.

If yours is a hospital HF program with a larger HF patient population and if you have dieticians, exercise physiologists, etc., on staff, a multidisciplinary model might suit your needs. For the private practice environment, a physician extender model is often the model of choice.

No matter which model is best suited to your situation, your choice will also need to consider the personality of the physician champion. In my experience, a mismatch between the model of care chosen and the personality of the program's medical director is rarely successful. This being said, in the right circumstances, a successful HF program can use any of the described models described above. The most common choice, though, is the physician extender or case manager models.

Once you select a model that suits your needs, you may not be able to commit the financial or staffing resources to develop the model you want. Take heart; all of these models of HF care benefit patients. As I suggested above, a new program might start with a physician champion concentrating on the HF patients in a given practice into an HF clinic. As the patient cohort grows, protocols and treatment algorithms can be developed to allow physician extenders to leverage the scarce physician resource. This can eventually evolve into a case manager approach as the growth of the program demands. The important step is to begin a systematic approach to your HF patients; i.e., develop an HF program. The rest will come.

Summary

The choice of healthcare delivery system you select will have important ramifications for how you interact with patients and how patients interact with your program. This decision will also determine how comprehensive the services of your program can be and how much the program can grow. In traditional models, the physician's time is the growth-limiting resource. In the physician extender, multidisciplinary team, and nurse case manager models, staff size and the physical facilities become the resources limiting the growth and scope of the program. These more complex models necessitate a more highly trained and autonomous staff, even when treatment is delivered via protocols. As the program leader, you must decide how much control over day-to-day operations you feel must rest in your hands and how comfortable you are in delegating important clinical decision making to others. If your program is to grow, however, it will need a model of care to accommodate that growth.

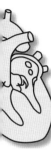

CHAPTER 5

First steps: a global view of the financial projections for your heart failure program

Your HF program needs to be run in a fiscally responsible way to be sustainable. Your decision to proceed with your program development will depend on the decisions you have made in your business plan. In this chapter, we will look at some strategic considerations that go into your financial projections. Some aspects of estimating your overhead and your projected revenue are straightforward; others depend on the scope of the HF program you envision. Important decisions on billing and staffing follow from your clinical approach to HF care. Different approaches require different infrastructures.

Specialized programs in a practice are developed for a number of reasons. A prevention program (i.e., a lipid clinic) is often launched because it increases the level of care that a practice provides in aggressively treating risk factors for coronary heart disease. It is a program that patients enjoy because of the increased attention they receive, and it is a method to attract patients to the practice and retain the patients once they have joined the practice. It is unusual for a prevention program to become a profit center for a practice.

An HF program also increases the level of care for patients with HF, and patients again enjoy the increased attention that they receive. Unlike a prevention program, however, an HF program should be a profit center for your practice. The approach described in this book is a volume-driven approach. To assure a financially viable program, some strategic decisions will need to be made before you open your doors regarding the projected size of your HF population, billing strategies, management of overhead, etc. In this chapter, we will examine the factors that should be considered to provide a clear pathway to profitability for your program.

Creating a disease management program in the current health-care environment

There is little question that, with the tools provided in this book, you can develop an HF center that provides a higher level of care than patients receive in the "usual care" situation. The program of intensive education followed by intensive monitoring of patient responses, coupled with sophisticated diagnostic testing and aggressive titration of medical and nonmedical therapies will result in better clinical outcomes.

Today, however, this is only half of the equation. One must not only provide superior clinical outcomes, but must also provide better clinical outcomes at a lower cost to be truly attractive to payors. This requires that a serious amount of energy be devoted to fiscal controls to keep your program financially on track. An HF disease management program utilizes intense education and monitoring to achieve its aims. This will clearly increase outpatient costs.

The premise is that a disease management program will reduce HF hospitalizations. The hospitalizations might also be shorter, since an outpatient HF program offering advanced services might be able to render most of the therapies a hospital would apply during the last few days of a typical HF hospital stay. If all this is true, then the increased outpatient costs are more than offset by reducing inpatient costs.

Controlling costs with a HF disease management program

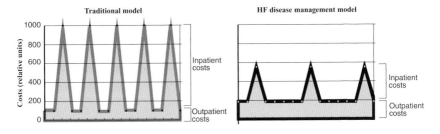

Disease management programs for HF can be successful in both the fee for service and capitated environments. Each environment has its own strengths and weaknesses. The fee for service environment rewards the practice that provides a broad scope of services and intensively monitors patients with diagnostic testing and therapeutic intervention. However, some services that are clearly helpful in reducing hospitalizations in HF patients, such as telemanagement, are not easily reimbursed in the fee for service environment.

On the other hand, capitated systems are often seen as healthcare at a discount, because incentives are in place that can encourage providers to provide fewer services for patients. In this environment, however, telemanagement would be viewed quite favorably, as it is a very cost-efficient way of monitoring a patient's progress.

In both payor environments, the philosophy is roughly the same. We spend $32 billion a year in the United States on HF, with the greatest portion being the cost of HF hospitalizations. Disease management programs can dramatically reduce the rate of HF hospitalizations. The fact that the intensified services of an HF center actually increase outpatient costs is more than outweighed by the impact that these programs have on inpatient costs.

Getting a handle on program costs

There are both fixed costs and variable costs that your HF center will have to evaluate. The fixed costs are going to be the rent, utilities, supplies, staff salaries, etc., that you will need to consider in operating a program. It can be difficult to decide how to assign fixed costs inside a complex physician practice or hospital. If the HF program is a freestanding facility, it is clear what the rent would be. If the program exists within a physical facility used by other parts of your practice or hospital, it can be problematic to assign various programs an appropriate portion of the costs of running an HF clinic.

If exam rooms are not run at capacity, for example, is the HF program to be "charged" for a given number of office hours a week in a given number of exam rooms, or is it to be charged simply for the number of exam room hours from office visits it actually uses? It can be a virtually impossible exercise to try to keep track of exactly what portion of the overhead should be assigned to the lipid clinic, which portion to the HF program, which portion to the clinical research program, etc.

A simpler approach is to calculate the total overhead of your practice, and then apply that overhead to all portions of the practice. This may not be fair but it is a simple and straightforward approach. If, for example, your practice overhead is 45%, then that 45% can be applied to all of the various programs within the practice. Again, this simple approach has its shortcomings, since not all programs have the same overhead. Such an overhead usually means that there is a heavy burden from the debt service on capital equipment such as nuclear cameras, 64-slice cardiac CT imagers, etc. A lipid clinic is not so resource intensive. However, this is a practical approach that I have found to be much more manageable than an attempt to track actual program costs on an ongoing basis. Counting paper clips can be a futile exercise.

Labor costs are usually the largest recurring cost of an HF program.

Variable costs are even more problematic. How much does an ECG really cost? What does it cost to schedule an appointment? Again, a simpler approach is to apply a fixed overhead rate to both the fixed and variable costs of your program.

Exceptions to the rule would likely be labor costs, usually the largest recurring cost of an HF program. In a resource intensive group of patients such as the HF patient cohort, there may be a higher nurse/patient ratio than there would be in an anticoagulation clinic. HF center-specific labor costs should be borne by HF center revenues. Shared labor costs (e.g., the practice receptionist) would be shared.

Likewise, capital equipment used exclusively by the HF center might need to be borne by HF revenues alone. An example of such capital equipment for the HF program might be noninvasive hemodynamic monitoring equipment or natriuretic peptide point of care testing equipment. Shared capital equipment (e.g., echocardiographic equipment or ECG machines) would be part of the 45% overhead figure mentioned above. Revenues attached to costs borne exclusively by the HF center would appropriately be unencumbered by that 45% tax. For example, revenues from noninvasive hemodynamic monitoring equipment might not have a 45% overhead applied; rather they would have the overhead attached to the service of the loans for that piece of capital equipment. Clearly, a sharp pencil is needed to control program costs.

Estimating sources of revenue

In a purely capitated environment, revenues are generally delivered on a per patient, per month basis. This can be a capitation rate for all the patients in a given patient population of a payor for which you are providing services. Alternatively, reimbursement can be based on a point of care capitation in which the per patient, per month capitation is paid only on patients who actually entered your HF program. The capitation rates for the latter situation are obviously going to be higher per patient (though for fewer patients) than for the former.

In the fee for service environment, the sources of revenue are going to be generated by diagnostic or therapeutic patient contacts. A common alternative scenario is a mixture of the two systems, where office visits are capitated, but certain patient services are paid on a pass through basis (e.g., infusion suite services), or where certain services are paid on a fee for service basis (e.g., echocardiograms or sleep apnea screening).

Since 80% of your revenues will come from the top 20 ICD-9 codes, use these 20 codes for projections of program revenues.

In either environment, one approach to determining what your revenues should be is to take the 20 most common procedures that you expect to be utilized by your HF patient population. If you multiply these 20 ICD-9 codes by the frequency that the service will be delivered to your patients, you can estimate the anticipated revenue necessary to care for your patient population each year. Since 80% of your revenues will come from the top 20 ICD-9 codes, some financial officers of HF programs use these 20 codes for their analysis and projections. In any case, during your first year these numbers will be approximate, but are surprisingly accurate. As time goes on and you gain program experience, your financial analysis should become more sophisticated.

Assigning "credit" for revenues

One problem that I have seen arise in HF programs is determining how revenues are credited within a practice. If, for example, the HF program generates a request for an echocardiogram as part of the benchmark testing for a patient and a physician not affiliated with the HF program reads the echo, who gets the credit? The HF program will want to receive credit so that it can justify its value to the partnership. The doctor interpreting the echo, however, did the work of interpretation, so he will want credit as well.

One solution that has worked well for me is to have a different color encounter form for each program within the practice. If an echocardiogram is ordered on a blue encounter form, it would represent activity from the HF clinic. If an echocardiogram is ordered on a yellow encounter form, it would represent activity from the research program. This way each program can be "credited" with the services that it provides and the revenue it generates. At the same time, the physician reading the echocardiogram can also receive the credit for reading the echo.

Who gets credit for services to HF patients and who gets the revenue are two different questions.

While on the one hand this appears to result in double counting of revenues of the practice, it at least captures the downstream revenues generated by the HF clinic so that the partnership can better evaluate the value of the program. If your program is losing $50,000 a month, you need to know that right away. If on the other hand you are generating $1,000,000 a year from your HF program without adding another partner to your practice, this needs to be recognized as well. Financial tracking can be challenging to recognize if the revenues have been buried in general practice revenues and the services performed by multiple providers in your practice.

In addition to the multicolored encounter forms, many computerized medical management systems have the ability to add modifiers to billing codes. If a blue encounter form is generated requesting an echocardiogram, when this code is recorded internally, it may be followed by a "- F" if the source of the service was the HF program. Likewise, it may have a "- R" following the ICD-9 code for services generated by the research program. These modifiers are not transmitted to the payors, but can be helpful for internal tracking of revenue flow.

Who gets "credit" for the services and who actually is allocated the funds for services delivered are two separate issues. The ways in which profits from revenues are divided in a practice is a very individual and often complex issue. Nonetheless, it is important for all the physicians in a practice to realize how much financial activity your HF program is generating, regardless of where the dollars end up within the practice.

Leveraging your growth-limiting resource with "incident to" billing

We have already discussed how, in most practices, the growth-limiting resource for your HF center will be the time and expense of physician services. By choosing a model of care such as a case manager model using physician extenders, that growth-limiting resource is leveraged.

Unless your case managers are all nurse practitioners or physician assistants, this strategy will require the use of "incident to" billing. The billing practices you will use in your program merit considerable attention as you set up and run your program. I cannot tell you how to bill for your services. Billing strategies are complicated by the ever-changing rules and strategies imposed by payors. Billing guidelines are often kept deliberately vague, so that the threat of penalty for incorrect billing will lead physicians to "under code" their services. If audited, there will not be any question that the billing strategies were within the guidelines if physicians bill less for their services than they should. However, with increasing downward pressure on physician revenues, the strategy of under coding becomes less and less attractive. Properly billing your services is a complex issue. Only you and your practice manager will be able to determine your billing practices, because only you and your practice manager will know the scope and intensity of the services you deliver to your patients.

Nowhere have I seen more confusion than in the area of "incident to" billing as I travel across the country. An "incident to" service is a service that is generated following an index visit with a physician. At the index visit, a physician may see a patient, provide a diagnosis for the patient, and then develop and initiate a treatment plan. "Incident to" visits are visits that are extensions of that index visit. "Incident to" services are provided not by the physician, but rather by an employee of the physician. A leased employee under the physician's direct control can also deliver "incident to" services. "Incident to" services are designed for the outpatient setting. The need to titrate so many medical therapies in an HF patient makes "incident to" billing a central strategy for the successful disease management program.

Nowhere have I seen more confusion than in the area of "incident to" billing as I travel across the country.

Only one "incident to" service can be provided on a given day, and "incident to" services must be under the direct personal supervision of a physician. This does not mean that the physician needs to be in the room with the healthcare provider providing the service. However, the physician must be on the premises of the office. He or she cannot be across the street making hospital rounds and simply be available by telephone. The physician must be available, should his or her services be needed while the care is delivered.

"Incident to" services can be provided by advanced practitioners, such as nurse practitioners or physician assistants. However, midlevel providers do not need to deliver the "incident to" services. Nurses or other healthcare providers can provide these services, as long as those providers are practicing within the scope of their professional license. In my opinion, using nurse practitioners for "incident to" services does not make sense. Midlevel providers or advanced practitioners can see patients on their own, without any need to rely on the physician index visit to initiate the "incident to" billing strategy.

Advanced practitioners in my opinion are better utilized as physician substitutes rather than physician extenders. An advanced practitioner has obtained further education and training in clinical assessment and physical diagnostic skills. When midlevel providers see a patient, this is not an "incident to" service. While the physician may still supervise this visit (and must supervise the visit if the service is to be billed as 100% of the Medicare allowable fee), such visits are not "incident to" a previous physician index visit. My nurse practitioners see patients independently and bill appropriately.

An example of an "incident to" service might be titration of ACE inhibitor therapy toward target doses of that drug.

An example of an "incident to" service might be titration of ACE inhibitor therapy toward target doses of that drug. The "incident to" visit can use any of the same E and M codes as a physician visit, yet typically are lower level visits, especially if not delivered by physicians or advanced practitioners. In my programs, "incident to" visits are usually protocol-driven visits with a low to moderate complexity of decision making.

When using "incident to" billing strategies, it is not necessarily the physician who performed the index visit who will bill for the subsequent services. If Dr Delgado sees a patient and decides to initiate a therapy that includes β-blocker titration, this index visit would generate a series of "incident to" visits. Two weeks later, during Dr Delgado's office hours a nurse may see the patient, assess the patient, and by written protocol, titrate therapy as appropriate. Since Dr Delgado is in the office seeing other patients, the "incident to" visit would be billed under Dr Delgado. Let's say that 2 weeks after that the patient returns for further titration, but the ordering physician (Dr Delgado) is now out of town. If his partner is in the office seeing patients, the visit can still take place, but the service would be billed under the second physician. It is the supervising physician who bills for the "incident to" services, not necessarily the physician who initiated the series of "incident to" visits.

While the same E/M billing codes used by the physician are also used for the "incident to" visit, it is unusual for an "incident to" visit to be billed out at a 99215 level. Most programs view "incident to" visits as simple visits rather than visits requiring such complex assessments and diagnostic skills as are implied by the 99215 billing code. On the other hand, some programs bill only 99211 visits for "incident to" visits. This has been called the "nursing code" because examples in the Medicare guidelines have stressed that a face-to-face contact with a physician is not necessary for 99211 visits. The billing for "incident to" visits, like any office visit, should reflect appropriately the level of complexity of these patient encounters. A drug titration may involve gathering patient symptoms on current therapy, assessing the patient's hemodynamics with a physical exam (and perhaps ancillary testing), and then making a clinical judgment as to whether the patient should have therapy up- or downtitrated, the size of the dose adjustment, and the mode of follow-up (telemanagement, clinic visit, etc.). These visits are protocol driven, but clinical judgment is still essential. This often goes beyond the scope of a 99211 visit. Certainly, if a physician, nurse practitioner, or physician assistant was providing this same service, the visit would be coded at a higher level of intensity than 99211.

An intriguing question that is as yet unanswered is whether telemanagement will become an "incident to" service.

An intriguing question that is as yet unanswered is whether telemanagement will become an "incident to" service. It is clearly more cost-effective to titrate medication (when possible from a safety standpoint) via the telephone rather than through an office visit. However, it is not clear when and whether such telemanagement will be considered an extension of the physician's index visit.

The current billing guidelines for Medicare suggest that telemanagement services should be bundled into the office visit. The office visit should then be billed accordingly, to reflect the extra effort and time required by the telemanagement contact, rather than have separate billing events for each telemanagement contact.

There are specific telemanagement codes (99371-99373), but in most states these are generally not reimbursed, and even when they are reimbursed, they are reimbursed at such a low level that the reimbursement does not justify the time and expense the practice expends on this activity.

I have also seen practices utilize the supervision of care codes (99374-99379) to obtain reimbursement for telemanagement of patients in nursing home facilities, hospice programs, and home health situations.

Again, your billing strategies can only be determined by you and your practice manager. You should strongly consider "incident to" practices, however, since this provides important leverage for your program to expand and give high quality, yet cost-efficient care.

Group visits

If you don't think that the "incident to" strategy will work for you, you can also consider using group visits to leverage physician time. If you are using a nurse practitioner for drug titration visits, group visits will leverage his or her time as well. This is a relatively new development that started in the western US a few years ago and has since spread throughout the country. There are two types of group visits used in HF programs.

If you are using a nurse practitioner for drug titration visits, group visits will leverage his or her time.

First, there is the drop-in group medical appointment (DIGMA). These are group visits for patients with an acute problem when the patient cannot or will not wait for an individual medical appointment. The group is run by the team of a prescribing healthcare provider (a physician, nurse practitioner, or physician assistant) plus a nurse (preferably with experience of running a group). This team sees a group of patients at once and deals with the acute problem during a 90-minute visit. Examples of such "urgent" problems might include a 10-lb weight gain over the weekend, the development of gynecomastia on spironolactone therapy, a change in anginal pattern, etc. HF is a dynamic disease. The DIGMA is a cost-efficient way to deal with the continual changes in status which HF patients face. Typically, the DIGMA strategy allows a clinician to triple the number of patients that can be seen in 90 minutes.

The second type of group visits began as the Community Health Continuity Clinic (CHCC) at the University of Colorado. Unlike the episodic care of the DIGMA groups, the CHCC provides continuity of care. A group of patients who enter your program at about the same time are subsequently seen as a group. In group visits, they receive basic education, but this is not a support group. It is a billable activity because care beyond education is given. For patients new to your program, this is the period of intense medication titration, and this can be done in a group setting for patients who waive HIPPA considerations, etc. While I was initially skeptical of this model, I have been pleasantly surprised that most patients will embrace it and find it a very positive experience. A series of four group visits can get most patients off to a great start in empowering our HF patients to get their arms around HF self-management.

I will further discuss the mechanics of group visits in a subsequent chapter. My point here is that the way you construct your infrastructure for patient flow will have an impact on your financial projections in that it impacts facility space, staffing needs, and billing philosophy. If "incident to" visits don't seem to fit in your environment, group visits are an alternative. However, this is not an either/or situation. I incorporate both methods in my HF programs to leverage our growth-limiting resource, which is physician time and expense.

Diagnostic and therapeutic procedures

In each program I have developed, the greatest financial challenge has been making the program profitable in its first year or two of operation. These critical first 2 years are a "honeymoon" period, during which it should be understood that start-up costs make achieving profitability especially difficult. Fixed costs such as staff salary need to be met immediately, whether or not they are supported by patient flow. However, some practices will demand early profitability. Certainly, if you can achieve a profit from the beginning, your program will be off to a great start.

A major difference between a lipid program and an HF program is the opportunity for an HF program to become self-sufficient early. This is because this chronic, lethal, incurable disease is also symptomatic. In addition, treatment of HF requires substantial diagnostic and therapeutic activity. Whereas in the lipid clinic the principal billable activity is blood work and medication adjustment two to four times a year, HF patients need continual monitoring to break the expensive cycle of hospitalization and rehospitalization that has traditionally characterized HF care. Projecting how many resources your HF population will consume is exactly that—a projection. There are some estimations that you can make.

An important part of the formula for program success we have already discussed is an early commitment from your program as to how you want you success to be judged. Some of the parameters you choose can be incorporated into benchmark visits where this data is collected. In fact, you might want to have the first benchmark visit before you even see the patient in your initial consult.

This preconsult visit could include a general health satisfaction questionnaire (e.g., the SF26) or a tool more specific to HF (e.g., the Minnesota Living with HF Questionnaire or the Kansas City Cardiomyopathy Questionnaire) to assess quality of life. We also use a questionnaire to get a baseline assessment for erectile dysfunction. In addition, we obtain responses to the Epworth and Berlin questionnaires to look for sleep disturbances. If your program accepts the data that 50% of HF patients have sleep apnea, you could even apply one of the home screening systems for sleep apnea such as the Respironics Stardust system or the Nexan Clearpath system. Your staff could measure functional status with a 6-minute-walk test and assess hemodynamics with a Cardiodynamics Bio-Z system. I also get a baseline assessment of patient knowledge of their disease with a questionnaire for later comparison with their knowledge level after being in our program for 6 months. At the preconsult visit, my staff assures that there is a recent ECG, echocardiogram, a platelet function assay for aspirin resistance, and a B-natriuretic peptide measurement before I see the patient at my initial consult. The benchmark visits will be repeated as separate visits at regular intervals (e.g., every six months). You will be able to use this data to identify gaps in the program's care and improve your services. The point here, though, is that all of this is generating billable activity. The infrastructure that you put in place before you open your doors will have important implications for running a fiscally responsible operation.

Beyond diagnostic activity are the therapeutic procedures that characterize HF care. Once devices such as biventricular pacing systems and defibrillators are implanted, it is likely that the device clinic (rather than the HF program) will follow the systems. However, these systems have crossed over into the realm of patient management. The Medtronic OptiVol system and the Guidant Latitude system track patient status, so the HF program should consider monitoring these systems in concert with the electrophysiologist. Further, cardiac resynchronization therapy (CRT) using biventricular pacemakers fail in 40% of HF patients. This has underscored the need to optimize the programming of CRT systems. This is not a one-time optimization at the time of implantation. As the heart remodels under the influence of the CRT system, the system needs to be reoptimized, perhaps as frequently as every 3 months. How to best optimize CRT systems is still in evolution. Newer echocardiographic equipment typically includes packages for this purpose, but this is a time-consuming procedure that doesn't easily fit into the flow of a busy echo lab. In addition, I would predict that payors will take a dim view of the routine use of echos every 3 months for CRT patients. More cost-effective alternatives have been proposed using the Cardiodynamics Bio-Z system and the Inovise Audicor system. These approaches do not require investment of precious physician time, and yet provide the same information on how to optimally program a CRT system.

I have never owned an external counterpulsation (ECP) system. However, this is a therapy that I have seen to have a significant impact on my HF patients when I referred them to ECP centers. The mildly positively results of the PEECH (Prospective Evaluation of Enhanced External Counterpulsation in Congestive Heart Failure) trial has led to a lukewarm response from payors to support ECP for HF patients in general. However, there is support for the patient with advanced refractory coronary heart disease, the most common etiology of HF in the United States.

It is important in your business plan to decide on the scope of your program. Your vision of who you are and who you are not as an HF program has profound implications for all subsequent decisions.

Current national guidelines take a dim view of chronic, scheduled outpatient infusions of inotropes. Certainly there is less need for this unproven option now that neurohormonal therapy has matured. Yet your HF program is going to routinely deal with the sickest of the sick. Many of the patients your staff will see every day could justifiably be hospitalized at each visit. An infusion suite is still an option to consider for your program for those patients, admittedly fewer in number, who transiently need an infusion of loop diuretics, vasopressin antagonists, nesiritide, and, yes, inotropes. Short-term inotropic support is still accepted in the United States by the medical community and by payors. For advanced HF patients, aggressive therapy will allow these patients to complete their time on earth at home rather than in the coronary care unit.

Another aggressive therapy that applies to a small number of patients is aquapheresis, an invasive method of removing water from the overloaded patient, similar to ultrafiltration. This is an expensive option for patients in your program with very advanced disease refractory to other approaches. Reimbursement is as yet unclear in the private practice situation. Hospital programs sometimes consider this therapy since it should be able to avoid hospitalizations, helping the hospital stop the hemorrhaging from DRG 127.

Summary

Only you can decide which services you want to offer. The point I am making here is that it is important in your business plan to decide on the scope of your program. Your vision of who you are and who you are not as an HF program has profound implications for all subsequent decisions. This thought process should begin in crafting your mission statement and guiding principles, and continue throughout your planning process. Once you decide how you are going to leverage your growth limiting resource, be it with "incident to" visits, group visits, etc. you can decide who you will use to perform these visits. Once you decide how you want your program's sucess to be assessed, you will know what measurements you want to make at benchmark visits. Once you decide on the scope of your program, you will know what sorts of services you will need to provide.

Your financial projections will follow from your planning decisions about the program that will best meet the needs of your patients, your practice/hospital, and your community. A common mistake is to try to do things the other way around. In the next chapter, we will go through the pro forma of a program that has a good chance of success.

CHAPTER 6

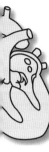

First steps: a heart failure program pro forma

Some HF programs succeed; others do not. Among the important decisions to make are the leadership of the program and the infrastructure to support that leadership and empower program staff to efficiently provide high-quality care. Here a pro forma of an HF program is presented that appears to have a good chance to be clinically successful and financially solvent early on.

Step one: assessing your patient population

The ACC/AHA HF guidelines encourage us to take a broad view of HF. Instead of waiting for symptoms to develop, the guidelines emphasize that the disease process begins with risk factors such as hypertension or diabetes (stage A HF). The process then advances to a phase where there has been a change in the structure of the heart but symptoms have not yet appeared (stage B HF). Once symptoms have appeared, whether they dissipate or not, the disease now has a different prognosis (stage C HF). Advanced HF is characterized as stage D. This scheme is meant to underscore the progressive nature of this disease. It supplements the New York Heart Association (NYHA) classification (Class I: no symptoms, Class II: symptoms with extraordinary activity, Class IIIA: symptoms with ordinary activity, Class IIIB: symptoms with minimal activity, Class IV: symptoms at rest). Since the NYHA classification is based on symptoms, it describes how a patient is doing at the moment, but not where they are in the overall natural history of their disease.

In either case, when you open your doors, it is unlikely that you will be referred a large cohort of asymptomatic or minimally symptomatic HF patients. You will be referred the sick HF patients who are difficult to manage and who consume a disproportionate share of healthcare resources. In my first HF program, most of the initial 100 patients had advanced HF:

NYHA class	No. of patients
I	0
II	9
III	62
IV	29

Virtually all patients in our initial population had advanced HF, with an average left ventricular ejection fraction of 22%. Surprisingly, even though the patients were referred by other cardiologists, the intensity of medical therapy was low:

Therapy	Baseline
ACEI/ARB	43
Digoxin	36
Diuretic	55
Triple therapy	21

Since this was in the mid-1990s, no patients referred were on β-blockers or aldosterone antagonists. Today I find this is still typical. If patients are referred on neurohormonal antagonists, it is usually on a non-evidence-based drug or on a subtherapeutic dose. Drug titration in a sick HF patient in the face of hypotension and HF symptoms is an art form. This is one of the main reasons that HF programs are needed. In our pro forma, one of the key components is the initial consult and medical follow-up. The follow-up will include physician visits, "incident to" visits, and group visits.

Physician revenues

What financial projections can we make regarding the HF care of these 100 patients during the first year that they are in the program? Let's begin with the revenues generated directly by the physician medical director with his or her own hands. Each HF patient entering the program will need an initial visit with the medical director. Coding for these visits would depend on the intensity and scope of services provided during the consult visit. In this pro forma, I project that the 91 patients in the first 100 referrals who had NYHA Class III/IV HF symptoms on presentation would have "level 5" (99245) consults, and the consults for the other 9 less-ill Class II patients would be "level 4" (99244). Revenues from these encounters would be:

Physician initial consults

Billing code	99245	99244	99243	99242	99241
Initial visit	91	9			
Medicare allowable	$213.41	$135.29	$115.13	$69.61	$31.76
Subtotal	$19,420.31	$1,217.61			
Total	$20,637.92				

Medicare allowable charges change from year to year, and what is covered is different from state to state. You will need to adjust the reimbursement numbers for your circumstances. The value of this pro forma exercise is to illustrate what you should include in your projections.

After the initial visit, the medical director will see the patients an average of once every few months, more often early in the year, less frequently as the year progresses. Let's project an average of four visits per patient in the first year. We can split the four visits per patient of Class III/IV patients evenly between level 4 (99214) and 5 (99215) visits. The four visits per patient for the Class II patients will be split evenly between level 3 (99213) and level 4 (99214) visits. These visits can be delivered by the physician or the midlevel practitioner. Most will probably be delivered by the physician, as this is the main point of patient contact for the physician. The physician visits are for issues best handled at the physician level.

These visits are often scheduled at a point appropriate for reassessment of a patient. For example, if at the initial consult certain goals were laid out (e.g., begin neurohormonal therapy with an angiotensin-converting enzyme (ACE) inhibitor, β-blocker, and an aldosterone antagonist and titrate by protocol to target doses), a physician visit should be set for the date at which titration would be complete. At that point in the patient's care it might be appropriate to assess the need for device therapy. On the other hand, if ACE inhibitor titration failed, the physician visit might be the point at which angiotensin receptor blockers (ARBs) or hydralazine/nitrate therapy would be considered.

Physician follow up visits

Billing code	99215	99214	99213	99212	99211
Office visit	182	254	18		
Medicare allowable	$112.25	$76.27	$48.65	$34.95	$19.47
Subtotal	$20,429.50	$19,372.58	$875.70		
Total	$40,677.78				

Physician revenues from the initial visit and follow-up office visits would total $60,934.61 in this pro forma. This is not going to be sufficient to support an HF program for 100 patients. Let us now examine the role of leveraging the physician resources of the program with a disease management program.

"Incident to" revenues

As mentioned in Chapter 5, each patient entering the HF program would have a preconsult visit or initial evaluation with the staff. This would include a number of baseline assessments through quality-of-life questionnaires, functional assessments with a 6-minute-walk test, noninvasive hemodynamic testing, etc. Beyond this testing, the preconsult visit includes a dietary evaluation, orientation to telemanagement and case managers, education about fluid and sodium budgets, a review of patient medications, obtaining medical records from other sources as necessary, and so on.

At this point in the pro forma, we will consider the evaluation and management (E and M) codes from this visit and not the procedure codes (from the 6-min walk, etc.). The complexity and scope of this visit is high. The visit takes significant time to complete. This is an appropriate visit to utilize an advanced practitioner in your program. In this pro forma, the scope and intensity of the services involved with the preconsult visit would be coded 99214.

Initial staff evaluation

Billing code	99215	99214	99213	99212	99211
Medicare allowable	$112.25	$76.27	$48.65	$34.95	$19.47
No. of visits		100			
Total		$7,627.00			

Our patient has now had a preconsult with the staff and an initial consult with the physician. Usually the next step is optimizing the medical regimen, especially the neurohormonal antagonists. We can start with ACE inhibitor therapy. Now recall that only 43 of our initial 100 patients were on ACE inhibitor therapy. For this pro forma, the other 57 patients will be started on ACE inhibitor during the initial consult and will require an average of two subsequent "incident to" titration visits (making 114 follow-up visits). In addition, let's assume that one-half of the 43 patients who came to us on an ACE inhibitor will need one titration visit to optimize therapy (22 more follow-up visits).

We can assume 10 patients will not tolerate an ACE inhibitor and will need two visits to initiate and titrate ARBs or the hydralazine/nitrate combination (20 follow-up visits). This brings the total to 156 follow-up visits for ACE inhibitor/ARB optimization.

As I have traveled the country, I have seen little consenus on how these visits are coded. I recall a practice that felt that all HF patients in their program were so sick and decision making in these patients was so complex that every visit supported a 99215 code. This seems a little excessive to me, and if nurses are delivering these "incident to" visits in your program, such a high level of coding may be beyond the scope of practice of a nurse. If nurse practitioners (NPs) or physician assistants provide these visits, then they really aren't "incident to." Midlevel providers can practice independently with physician supervision. They don't require the physician index visit to start a plan of care.

Other programs feel that if a nurse provides a service, it must be billed 99211. This is certainly safe, but I don't think that it reflects the scope and intensity of services provided. Even though drug titration visits are using protocol-driven therapy, nurses are using substantial clinical judgment when adjusting therapy in these sick patients. A 99211 level of billing does not seem appropriate. After considerable discussion and consultations (with conflicting advice) we decided that these visits should be coded 99212. Projected revenues from ACE inhibitor titration in our 100 patients will be:

ACE inhibitor/ARB hydralazine-nitrate therapy

Billing code	99215	99214	99213	99212	99211
Office visit				208	
Medicare allowable	$112.25	$76.27	$48.65	$34.95	$19.47
Total	$5,452.20				

None of the patients in this pro forma presented on β-blocker therapy. The titration schedule for β-blockers is less predictable than for ACE inhibitors. Many hemodynamically fragile patients need half-step titrations or may need to even be downtitrated once or twice on the way to target doses. Other patients with hypertension can be initiated at a higher dose than the typical starting doses. For this pro forma, I project that these patients will need four visits on average for β-blocker initiation and titration.

β-blocker titration visit protocols often involve more patient education (the timing of doses, whether to take with food, spacing doses from other hypotensive agents, etc.) and evaluation of patient status before moving on to the next dose level. However, the frequent vital signs and prolonged observation in the office that were previously required after each and every dose change are no longer considered necessary. Despite the increased intensity of β-blocker titration visits, to be conservative we will still use level 99212 coding for these visits.

β-blocker therapy

Billing code	99215	99214	99213	99212	99211
Office visit				400	
Medicare allowable	$112.25	$76.27	$48.65	$34.95	$19.47
Subtotal				$13,980.00	
Total	$13,980.00				

None of the 100 patients were on aldosterone antagonists. As the only agent specifically tested in HF patients, spironolactone would be initiated in all 100 patients. We can assume an average of two visits per patient for drug initiation and up- or downtitration and monitoring of blood potassium. With an 8% incidence of gynecomastia, we can project eight additional visits in the 100 patient cohort to convert the affected patients to eplerenone.

I have already made the point that careful monitoring of potassium levels is important with aldosterone antagonist therapy. I have not included the revenues from lab draws for this monitoring. I have also not included the billing for telemanagement of potassium levels. In the last chapter, I discussed how we are directed to bundle this monitoring into the E and M codes for patient visits, increasing the billing level to reflect the increased scope of a visit that includes subsequent patient contacts by phone. If your program will provide lab services or telemanagement, you should include these activities in your pro forma.

These issues are handled differently by different HF programs I have seen. Again, it is not my intent to present the most aggressive billing strategy open to your program. I do want to lay out the options for you, but I want to keep this pro forma conservative. My hope is that even with a conservative approach, you will see a path that your HF program can follow to build a financially sound program. We will therefore put into this pro forma an average of two visits per patient for aldosterone antagonist titration.

Spironolactone therapy

Billing code	99215	99214	99213	99212	99211
Office visit				208	
Medicare allowable	$112.25	$76.27	$48.65	$34.95	$19.47
Total	$7,269.60				

Some patients will decompensate during the year and come in for an unscheduled visit. According to Medicare, the typical HF patient decompensates 1.3 times a year. A common instance of this is when a patient has sodium and fluid indiscretions over several days and comes into the office volume overloaded. Therapy will need to be adjusted. Services at these visits will be provided by the physician or a midlevel provider. However, these unscheduled visits may well become the index visit for a subsequent series of "incident to" follow-up visits. Returning to our volume-overloaded patient, during the unscheduled visit it is likely that loop diuretics will be added or increased. Perhaps metolazone will be added for a short-term as well. "Incident to" visits will then be scheduled to follow-up on the patient's response to this change in therapy and to further adjust or stop the short-term intervention according to protocol. We will call these follow-up visits "special visits" in this pro forma.

Coupled with visits for medical nutrition therapy and ongoing monitoring of patient progress via the benchmark data collection visits (repeat quality-of-life assessments, 6-min walks, etc.), special visits would average four visits per patient per year.

Special visits

Billing code	99215	99214	99213	99212	99211
Office visit				400	
Medicare allowable	$112.25	$76.27	$48.65	$34.95	$19.47
Subtotal				$13,980.00	
Total	$13,980.00				

You will note that I have not included group visits specifically in the pro forma. These visits are billable, and nearly all of the new patients that are referred to my program go through a set of four group visits to begin to understand their disease and to start the titration of their medical regimen. I would need to subtract four of the titration visits listed above to include the CHCC (Community Health Continuity Clinic) group visits. It is only for simplicity that I have left them out. The impact is revenue neutral. The value of group visits is that it leverages your staff time. More patients can be seen in less time without any sacrifice in the quality of care when group visits are used. The DIGMA (drop-in group medical appointment) group visits are harder to quantitatively project, as the size of the group attending the DIGMA group meetings is not constant. They could be estimated in the Special Visits section, but I am trying not to overstate the case for the viability of an HF program with a complex argument.

In your business plan, it is prudent for you to underpromise so that your program can overdeliver. Painting a rosy scenario with unrealistic expectations for patient volumes and program revenues sets you up to fail to meet expectations, which you will then have to explain to a disappointed group of partners or hospital board. It is much more pleasant to report that your program is running ahead of projections.

It is understandable that you are enthusiastic about your program's prospects. Otherwise, you would not be spearheading this effort. I would argue that you need to curb your enthusiasm when assembling your financial projections. Further, overpromising is unnecessary. Even in this conservative pro forma, "incident to" billing leverages physician resources, increasing revenues by 40% over the revenues resulting from physician visits alone.

Total physician-generated revenue		"Incident to" revenue	
Initial visits	$20,256.83	Initial evaluation	$7,627.00
Office visits	$40,677.78	ACE inhibitor/ARB	$5,452.20
Total	$60,934.61	Spironolactone	$7,269.60
		Beta blockade	$13,980.00
		Special visits	$13,980.00
		Total	$48,308.80
Physician revenue		$60,934.61	
"Incident to" revenue		$48,308.80	
Total		$109,243.41	

The catch: program expenses

The E and M services provide just over $1000 per patient. This is a nice start. This is more than you could expect from a lipid program, for example. No doubt, though, you will be quick to point out that while revenues are nice (without them your program will clearly fail), they need to be viewed through the prism of overhead expenses. Just as we discussed in the last chapter, your costs will be heavily influenced by the scope of services that you want to provide and how you want to provide them. Physicians are more expensive than NPs. Nurse practitioners are more expensive than nurses. If you use an NP to deliver "incident to" services, it will require more patients in your program to reach your breakeven point. Again, I use NPs as physician substitutes, not physician extenders. A reasonable first cut at costs for an HF program could be:

Program costs: fee for service environment	
Administrative costs	$20,000.00
1/4 MD, 1 NP, 2 RNs	$200,000.00
Facility/supplies	$30,000.00
Breakeven point	$250,000.00

E and M codes are not enough to sustain the program, but they get you more than halfway. You should conclude from this that either you can't expect to break even until you have more than 250 HF patients in your program, or you need to look beyond E and M codes alone. The first place to look is the diagnostic testing and the therapeutic procedures that are part of an HF program. Such activity begins with the preconsult visit and continues as long as the patient is in the program.

Diagnostic testing

During the preconsult visit, I have suggested that the baseline assessments include some procedures. For example, home screening for sleep apnea could be reasonably applied. Among the available systems is the Clearpath system from Nexan. Reimbursement varies severalfold for this testing from state to state. Florida supports this testing at the low end of the range of reimbursement. To be conservative, let's use that level of payment for this pro forma. The available evidence tells us that half of the patients tested will have abnormal test results. Even if only a quarter of the patients tested were found to have abnormal results, it would still be worth testing all of your patients. These patients can then be referred to a sleep lab, or handled however you handle sleep apnea in your practice.

Sleep apnea testing is only done during the initial evaluation of your patients. The same is true for most patients you test for aspirin sensitivity. Most other procedures in your program will be done periodically. During both the preconsult visit and benchmark visits patients will undergo other tests repeatedly, such as a 6-minute-walk test, noninvasive hemodynamic testing (e.g., with the Cardiodynamics Bio-Z system), and a measurement of B-natriuretic peptide levels. If we assume that 20% of patients sick enough to be referred to an HF program require cardiac resynchronization therapy, then you might include quarterly optimization of the system with the Inovise Audicor system (again, trying to reduce the costs that would come from the use of echocardiography for this purpose). For our purposes here we can assume that these procedures will be done twice a year. The staff will probably utilize Bio-Z and B-natriuretic peptide testing more frequently than the physician. A cardiologist has extensive training in cardiology and will need less support to assess a patient. Others with less training often find ancillary testing helpful to confirm or guide their decision making. I will again be conservative in this pro forma. Downstream revenues will also include echocardiograms to monitor the course of disease and reverse remodeling. Routine echocardiograms are not mandated by current HF guidelines. They may or may not be part of the benchmark parameters by which you want your program to be judged.

A conservative estimate for diagnostic testing for 100 patients during their first year in an HF program is $173,117. Between the E and M codes for office visits and the diagnostic testing, we have now crossed the breakeven point. One hundred patients will make your program a sustainable effort.

Therapeutic procedures

In the last chapter, I touched on the utility of infusion therapy and external counterpulsation. These are expensive therapies and need to be applied judiciously. Because they require advanced skills and monitoring, reimbursement levels, even after recent reductions, are good. If these services are a part of your program, then your program will be profitable in its first year even with 100 patients, as shown in the example below. Further, with a staff of one-fourth of a physician, one NP, and two RNs (registered nurses), your program could handle considerably more than 100 patients without adding additional staff.

Other approaches

Another approach is to look at the HF activity is to use the relative value units (RVUs) your practice expended in the last year on HF services as a guide to how busy your program will be initially. Of course, it is unlikely that all the partners in your practice will refer all of their HF patients to

Total physician-generated revenue		Ancillary revenue	
Initial visits	$20,256.83	"Incident to"	$48,308.80
Office visits	$40,677.78	Diagnostic testing	$173,117.00
Subtotal	$60,934.61	Infusion services	$35,550.00
		ECP	$122,323.60
		Subtotal	$379,299.40
Physician revenue		$60,934.61	
Ancillary revenue		$379,299.40	
Total program revenue		$440,234.01	

your program, so you need to anticipate what is reasonable portion of the practice HF patients will come your way. Nonetheless, armed with the number of HF patient population that you can expect in your practice, the number of visits these patients generated, and the number of RVUs expended on those visits, your financial forecasting is well on its way.

Knowing how much revenue came from these HF patients and the number of RVUs expended, you can determine the number of RVUs you need per year to care for an HF patient in your practice. Applying the Medicare reimbursement per RVU gives you a means of evaluating contracts you are offered (especially capitated contracts) for HF care.

Further, knowing the revenues that came from your HF patients over the last year, if you apply your average practice overhead percentage to these revenues, you can determine the cost of caring for an HF patient for a year in your practice.

The costs of a formal HF program will be different than the traditional model of care your practice used in previous years. So will the revenues. The RVU analysis can be a useful way to determine where your practice is now so that you can compare that starting point to where you think your program will be at the end of its first year of operations.

What about year 2?

Your patients will find the first year in your program to be the most intense. That is when the most education needs to be done, and when the bulk of drug initiation and titration will be done. In the first year of therapy, we feel it is very important to "touch" our new HF patients very frequently to fully introduce ourselves to the patient and to give the patient a clear idea of what to expect from the program. Subsequent years require less and less contact.

After the first year, your program will focus on further education and reeducation, followed by chronic monitoring. There will be periods of increased therapeutic activity when a patient decompensates or when a new event such as a myocardial infarction occurs.

Your HF program will depend on the growth of your patient population to support your effort. This should not be a problem since HF is so prevalent, but a portion of your program resources will need to be devoted to establishing and maintaining referral sources to achieve long-term success. The financial projection of your business plan will probably attempt to see 3 years into the future. These days, that is no easy task. Patient sources, reimbursement levels, overhead costs are neither constant nor dependable. Flexibility and a willingness to embrace change will be a part of the successful HF program.

Summary

There are many reasons to establish an HF program. Your program will give you the professional satisfaction of doing a better than average job for your patients. Your program should establish your practice as a center of excellence in the treatment of HF. There is no reason, though, that your HF program should not ultimately be a profit center for your practice. The first months or years may be difficult financially as the program grows to a critical size, and as you develop your protocol and treatment algorithms—your "style." Different styles will require different infrastructures. Your business plan should anticipate revenues and costs of the E and M activity as well as the diagnostic testing and therapeutic interventions you choose to include in your program. Ultimately, though, your program should represent an alternative source of revenue for your practice in the face of continued downward pressure on traditional sources of medical revenue for medical services.

Assembling the pieces of your program

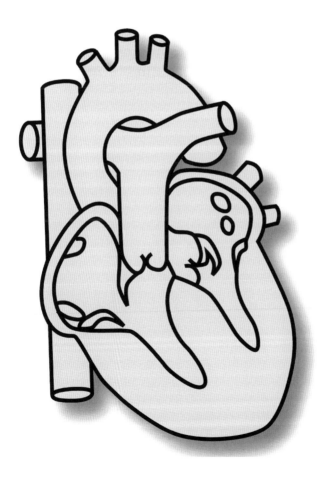

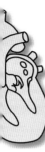

CHAPTER 7

Assembling the pieces: the managers of your program

The management of a successful heart failure program most easily rests on the shoulders of a physician medical director, who serves as the champion of the program internally and is the face of the program to the community. The heart and soul of the program, though, often emanates from the clinical director, who runs day-to-day operations. Your management team will also include support from the practice or hospital administrator. Other management structures may also be superimposed on this basic management team. The success of the program, though, depends on this basic management triad.

Step one: the physician champion

I have already laid out the critical role that I feel is played by the physician champion of an HF program. A program can be successful without the physician champion, but this is a challenging task. The unsuccessful HF programs that I have seen over the last 10 years are often characterized by a practice or hospital turning to a midlevel provider who is directed to "start an HF program."

In these circumstances, HF care is seen as a simple matter of a little straightforward patient education coupled with placing patients on whatever therapy the Joint Commission on Accreditation of Healthcare Organizations or the Agency for Healthcare Research and Quality decrees. These standards lag not only state-of-the-art care, but also national guidelines. A simple example is the standard that ACE (angiotensin-converting enzyme) inhibitor therapy is mandated for HF patients, but not β-blocker therapy. This standard lags behind current national guidelines, which give the highest level of recommendation to β-blocker therapy, but more importantly to clinicians, it lags our evidence from clinical trials on the value of β-blockers in HF by over a decade. A committed physician champion no doubt would insist on the use of evidence-based β-blocker therapy for the HF patients in the program.

The medical director determines the short- and long-term goals of the HF program, sets the policies and procedures that the program will follow, trains the staff, develops the treatment algorithms, and sets the program on its way to success. My HF programs have only become successful once everyone bought into a uniform treatment style. While it is important to customize therapy to each HF patient, there is a style to how your program will approach the lifestyle changes, medical therapy, and long range goals you offer your patients. In my programs, we are aggressive in some ways, conservative in others. Other programs give equally good HF care, but have their own style. Your medical director will develop your program's style.

The medical director determines the short- and long-term goals of the HF program, sets the policies and procedures that the program will follow, trains the staff, develops the treatment algorithms, and sets the program on its way to success.

Your HF program needs a champion. HF programs are still relatively new, and you can anticipate that your staff will meet some resistance as they do their jobs. The resistance will come from other physicians within and outside your practice. Resistance may also come from hospitals, from other staff, and even from some patients who are used to receiving all of their care from a physician.

As a good leader, the medical director will need to provide inspiration to the HF program staff. Esprit de corps is important in any new endeavor; your staff must believe they are delivering care that is superior to that which their patients can obtain elsewhere in your community. Your medical director is an important source of that feedback and encouragement.

There will be battles to fight for your program. There will be battles with the hospital, with your partners, with insurance carriers, and so on. The medical director must bear the brunt of these battles and shield the staff so that they are free to concentrate on patient care.

The medical director must also lead the program to remain current in its approach to HF care. There is no cure for this disease, so it is not surprising that treatment is constantly in a state of flux. Ongoing quality of care improvement and ongoing refinement of treatment algorithms generally falls to the medical director. It is up to the physician champion to evaluate these new therapies and decide which ones are appropriate for your HF program.

Most important of all, perhaps, is the medical director's responsibility to demonstrate to the patients that they are in a program of the highest quality. HF is a complex lethal disease. Patients in an HF program must feel not only that they are in the hands of an expert team, but also that they are benefiting from the knowledge and experience of a physician with a special interest in HF and his or her team of HF experts.

Step two: the clinical director

While the medical director is the champion of your program, the heart and soul of a program is that special asset who serves as the clinical director. In my experience, this role has been filled by physician assistants, nurse practitioners, RNs, and BSNs. I have found that there is little relationship between the initials following the name of the clinical director and the suitability of that manager to meet the requirements of the position. What is needed is someone who can get the best out of his or her staff. This has more to do with the person than the degree.

It is also important that there be a high degree of respect and trust between the medical director and the clinical director. An unwritten tenet of the models of healthcare delivery that we discussed in earlier chapters is that the key to the successful treatment of chronic diseases is to get the physician out of the business of performing all of the tasks associated with patient education, patient compliance, and HF prevention for which the physician is ill-suited.

A critical requirement for physicians to be comfortable in relinquishing control of patient care is that patient care is left in competent hands.

Physicians may be hesitant to give up direct control of what is happening with their HF patients. A critical requirement for physicians to be comfortable in relinquishing that control is that patient care is left in competent hands. As opposed to the lipid clinic or Coumadin clinic, the clinical director of an HF program is assuming clinical responsibility for some of the sickest patients in a cardiovascular practice. The clinical director needs to be up to that task.

A problem that you will probably encounter during the search for a clinical director is that healthcare personnel with training in disease management are rare. I would advise you to expect a 6-month "training" period as your clinical director ramps up his or her skills. Clinical directors of HF programs I have met around the country come from diverse backgrounds, from critical care nursing to home health nursing, from clinical research to nursing administration. Skills from all of these backgrounds will prove valuable. None of these alone will be enough.

Knowing how to manage acute pulmonary edema in the coronary care unit does not prepare a nurse to manage chronic HF in the outpatient setting. The goals and principles of therapy in these two situations have little in common. A home health nurse tends to send patients with a significant change in symptoms to the emergency department. In an

HF program designed to avoid hospitalizations, this behavior must be unlearned.

It is not surprising, then, that it takes a while for a clinical director to grow into the job and to get comfortable with the tempo of both the disease and the therapy. For the first 6 months of the program, the medical director will also be the de facto clinical director. For long-term success, though, these two roles need to be separated. The strategy for success in HF programs is to leverage physician resources. A good clinical director provides that leverage.

Characteristics of an ideal clinical director

- Nurse, nurse practitioner, physician assistant—the degree matters less than the person
- Not just intelligent but intellectually curious and with a thirst for continual learning
- Good depth of clinical knowledge, both in HF and in medicine in general
- Interested in HF as a complex, chronic, and incurable disease
- Independent, self-motivating, and infectiously enthusiastic
- Good leadership skills
- Takes ownership in the program
- Organized and meticulous enough to follow protocols, produce good documentation, maintain the program database, and commit to outcomes research
- Good interpersonal skills with staff, patients, and referring physicians
- Good communication skills for education and public speaking
- Someone you can trust with the sickest patients in your practice

---

Your program will take on the personality of both the medical director and the clinical director. Your choice of the leadership of your HF program needs to be done carefully. Unless there is trust and chemistry between the medical director and clinical director, it will be difficult for the rest of the staff to become a team, and it will be difficult to instill confidence in the patients of the program. The bond between the two directors is important for your HF program to develop its treatment style.

Simply stated, I have found no substitute for a committed clinical director.

Step three: the administrator

The medical director and the clinical director focus on optimizing the medical care of the patients in your program. The practice or hospital program administrator organizes the resources of the practice or hospital in support of the HF program to meet its clinical goals. You will need good relations with payors to facilitate patient access to your program. Your new HF program will have physical facility requirements. The administrator can tackle these problems.

We have discussed that you will need to make some decisions about billing strategies. Front office support will also be required. The administrator is responsible for all of these functions. Just as important, the administrator will take the point position in seeking HF "carve out" contracts for your program from payors and for marketing your program to the medical and patient community.

The medical director, the clinical director, and the administrator charged with administering your program are all critical pieces of a successful HF program. I have seen programs succeed without one of these elements, but not if two of the team were absent.

Step four: oversight bodies

While the medical and clinical directors, along with the administrator, will set up and run your HF program, the program is often responsible to a larger body. In the private practice environment, the program must prove its value to the practice partnership. Hospital HF programs likewise will report to some form of oversight body. This could be made up of members of the hospital administration, the medical staff, or both. In either case, let's call this oversight body the executive committee.

The executive committee represents those who will refer patients to your program. Those referrals are the lifeblood of your program.

I have found it helpful as a medical director to prepare annual summaries of my HF programs' activities for the executive committee so that it is clear what the program has accomplished. In the midst of a busy clinical program, you and your staff may understand how the program is growing and the impact you are having on your patients' lives. Those outside the program may have no idea what you are doing or worse, may have a distorted and incorrect view. Being the champion of your program often means justifying your program at an executive committee meeting every month.

The executive committee is also helpful in providing an outside perspective for program operations. For example, including the executive committee in the formation of treatment algorithms and telemanagement protocols will make it clear upfront to the committee just how much clinical responsibility you are delegating to the program staff. If there is general agreement that your plans and activities are reasonable, then you are on the right track. If there are serious objections, then your program may be embracing a strategy that won't be accepted in the community. The executive committee represents those who will refer patients to your program. Those referrals are the lifeblood of your program. Though you may not agree with some of the opinions of the committee, you do need to consider these opinions seriously.

The executive committee's role is to help with strategy. Group leadership doesn't lend itself well to day-to-day operations. The style of HF care the program delivers will reflect the approach of the medical and clinical directors. For example, the executive committee usually controls the overall budget of the program, but doesn't do the hiring and firing of staff. The medical director will decide if the program should include an infusion suite, but the executive committee may need to find the space and approve the funds for the infusion chairs, etc.

HF program management structure

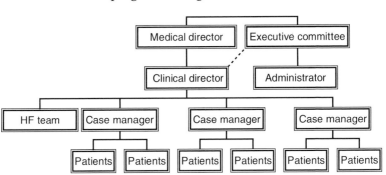

Summary

The management of your HF program will likely fall into three sets of hands. The physician champion who serves as the medical director will provide the vision and driving force for the program. The clinical director will provide the day-to-day culture, or heart, of the program. An administrator is charged with the essential financial support for the program.

With these three elements, your HF program is well on its way to success. These three leaders need to talk often as the program is formed and should meet periodically thereafter to maintain success. The program may also report to an oversight body such as an executive committee. In the hospital setting, the executive committee might consist of all physicians in the community who might be interested in HF care. This committee often controls the purse strings of the program and oversees the activities of the HF program. One does not want a committee to run the program in microscopic detail, though, or the program is likely to fall prey to the phenomenon of "paralysis by analysis," whereby even the simplest decisions become difficult. The program needs to trust the leadership of the medical and clinical directors, with the oversight of the executive committee assuring that all interested parties have a stake in the program's success.

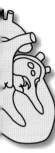

CHAPTER 8

Assembling the pieces: the front line staff

While management staff is critical to program success, this by no means implies that the rest of the program's staff is somehow unimportant. There is plenty of work to go around, and the personnel who interface with the patients on a day-to-day basis become the human face of the program. These are the personnel who convey the impression of the competence of your program. In disease management programs, the voice on the phone doing the telemanagement and the case manager arranging resources and adjusting therapy will have much more contact with the patient than the medical director.

More than once, the growth of my HF program has slowed to a stop, not because of a loss of managers, but because of the loss of one or two front line staff. HF therapy can be "high tech," with sophisticated diagnostic testing and therapeutic interventions. Disease management programs, though, are a "high touch" approach to HF therapy, with frequent patient contacts to educate patients about their disease and to increase compliance to therapy. Who does the touching is very important.

In every HF program I have established, in fact in every disease management program I have established, be it a lipid program, an HF program, or whatever, the patients in the program quickly become attached to the staff. This is something I not only support but also foster. Part of the reason I find the preconsult visits useful is that during that visit, patient education about sodium and fluid budgets, and self-management strategies for loop diuretic therapy are discussed with the patient. This establishes the staff in the patient's mind as a competent source of information relating to their HF. Before they see me for the first time, the patient experiences firsthand that the program is a center of HF expertise. Likewise, when I first see the patient, I am accompanied by that patient's case manager. At the end of the history and physical, I ask the case manager what he or she sees as the next therapeutic intervention we should make. This way, the patient sees my confidence in the staff. This establishes that when the case manager speaks, it is with my authority. It also makes it clear that the case manager is part of the team and that I am not "dumping" the patient onto the staff when subsequent visits do not include me. If, as I suggest, there are four nonphysician visits for every physician visit, the patient needs to see the staff as a reliable source of care.

In every disease management program I have established, the patients in the program quickly become attached to the staff.

Finding the staff for your program is not a simple task. Unless your staff is recruited from another HF program, there is little opportunity for your future staff to obtain the necessary skill set. The establishment of the American Association of Heart Failure Nurses may change this in the coming years. For now, though, I often see program recruiters turn to critical care nurses as the best candidates. This is a good source, but keep in mind that critical care nurses are attuned to the short-term needs of very ill patients. What you need is a critical care nurse with the personality of a home health nurse who cares for patients over the long-term.

Whatever the source of your staff, it will be up to the medical director and clinical director to train this staff. As one of my HF nurses told me, "you don't know what you don't know." Most medical nurses feel they know how to take care of HF. Most likely they have taken care of hospitalized HF patients. They might not be prepared, though, for the ambulatory NYHA Class IIIB patient who presents with a systolic BP of 96 mm Hg and a creatinine of 2.3 mg/dL who needs further drug titration. These patients could be justifiably hospitalized at each visit. Training your staff to care for these ill patients on an outpatient basis is up to you.

As with your choice of your program's clinical director, you are looking for front line staff who are the sort of intelligent, independent thinkers in whom you can entrust the day-to-day decisions that characterize the ongoing care of your HF patients. Again, in a "high touch" program, who does the touching is important.

Case managers

The nurse practitioners, physician assistants, or nurses who serve as your case managers are the main point of contact between the patient and your program. The case manager stands beside the patient at the center of the wheel, with spokes extending out to the various other specialists and services available to the patient, such as physical therapists, home health nurses, and dieticians.

Case managers are the patient advocates, assuring that patients do not get lost in the labyrinth of a large cardiology group or hospital. As practices grow and physician–patient time is pressured, there is a risk that the patient begins to feel like a number, or "just another case." The case manager rehumanizes the treatment process. We can only treat patients one at a time. The case manager assures that care in your HF program is individualized.

The qualities of a good case manager include medical competence, the intellectual capacity to apply protocol-driven therapy with some independence, and a real interest in HF and the special needs of this chronically ill, complex, and incurable patient cohort. It is essential that the case manager has the compassion needed to deliver not just medical therapy, but patient care.

Case managers will need to endlessly educate and monitor the patients in their charge. There is a fine line between the patience needed to instruct Mr Jones for the 37th time about his fluid and sodium budgets and the risk of making Mr Jones dependent on the case manager for every decision. It is difficult for case managers not to get attached to their patients. At times, case managers need to give "tough love" to help train patients to be in charge of their own disease management.

The number of case managers you will need depends upon your case mix.

The number of case managers you will need depends upon your case mix. Disease management companies (who are basically vendors of telemanagement) will have pods of hundreds of patients per case manager. In my experience, there have been times when several sick patients in a pod have made it difficult for a case manager to handle more than 25–50 clients. If there are a large number of NYHA Class I and II patients in your program, e.g., a large number of patients with asymptomatic left ventricular dysfunction, patient pods can be large. When your program starts, it is likely that only NYHA Class III and IV patients will be referred, so pods must be smaller.

Similarly, as the experience of your case manager grows, his or her pods can be larger. During the first few months of a new case manager's employment, you will be educating him or her about the pathophysiology of HF, the rationale behind your treatment algorithms and protocols, the policies and procedures of your program, etc. Pods need to be small during this training period. When the case managers are taking call, they need to be strong enough in their knowledge base to know when to follow treatment protocols and when to go to the next level in the chain of command (namely to the clinical director or the medical director) with their questions.

Heart failure clinic staff

Whenever possible, my HF nurses see patients along with me in the HF clinic. This way, they hear firsthand the teaching I do with the patients about the rationale for β-blocker therapy, or the optimization of ACE (angiotensin-converting enzyme) inhibitor therapy, or when a patient should combine two different types of diuretics. This helps the staff reinforce my education efforts by sending a consistent message. The HF staff also hears whether patients can (or cannot) tell me their fluid and sodium budgets or their dry weight. The staff can observe firsthand whether the patient is absorbing what we have taught him. By doing clinic visits together with my staff, the patient then identifies the staff member with the program and with me. We have learned the new math of patient education I discussed before: $7 \times 1 = 0$ and $3 \times 3 = 2$. Again, if you teach a patient seven things once, they likely will remember nothing. If, on the other hand, you teach the same thing three times, most patients will absorb two of the three messages.

The HF clinic nurse can supplement the case manager as a point of patient contact.

Case managers see patients with me as well, but as their pod grows, they have less time available for clinic activities. The HF clinic nurse can supplement the case manager as a point of patient contact. If you start a patient on spironolactone, the clinic nurses arrange for potassium monitoring. If you initiate β-blocker therapy, they arrange the titration visits, etc. Written protocols guide the HF clinic nurse in these activities. Examples of such protocols can be found later in this book.

The clinic nurses are LPNs (licensed practical nurses) and RNs (registered nurses). The main quality these nurses must have is a desire to learn about HF and a desire to form the sort of relationship with HF patients that will be necessary long-term to carry out our program of education, treatment, and monitoring. Much of the educational reinforcement comes from the clinic nurses. They will attend the patient group visits. They may well teach some of the group classes you might offer the public. These nurses are the glue that makes the program hang together as a whole.

Dietary services

The question of whether you acquire a dietician depends on how your program is set up in your business plan. I have operated HF programs with and without a full-time dietician. I have found the services of a dietician to be important. Sodium and fluid budgets are important to HF therapy, but so are controlling other risk factors for atherosclerosis and myocardial ischemia. Since lifestyle modification is one of the safest and most effective therapies for atherosclerosis and HF, I have found a full-time dietician to be helpful. He or she is better trained than I am to give practical advice to patients on dietary strategies and therapeutic lifestyle changes. However, financial realities might dictate that your program cannot have full-time dietary services. In a start-up program, you may want to contract with a hospital dietary department or with an independent dietician part time to arrange these services.

Summary

Only you can decide what personnel you need to staff your HF program. Who you need depends on the scope of services you want to provide. I can only tell you that HF programs I have developed were best suited for a clinical director, one to two RNs, one to two LPNs, and a full- or part-time dietician to manage a population of 500 HF patients. The HF programs I describe here are volume driven and leverage physician resources by having four contacts with the nonphysician HF staff for every physician visit.

Finding the right people around whom you will build your program is difficult but crucial. Nurse case managers and HF clinic staff have the most contact with the patients in your program. They are the patient interface of your program. As medical director, you must train this staff and assure that they provide HF care the way you want it to be delivered and that their caseload is appropriate for their abilities. These abilities may change over time. Some of the ancillary staff needs can be outsourced if your program is small. Again, your overall staffing needs reflect the scope of services your HF program has decided to provide.

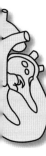

CHAPTER 9

Assembling the pieces: the physical facility

The physical layout of your heart failure (HF) program can be modest, but should include exam rooms for the HF clinic, group and/or individual education areas, a telemanagement office, and front- and back-office support space. As with staffing issues, the physical needs of your HF program depend upon the scope of the program, the size of the patient population served, and the treatment style you have selected to care for your patients. For example, you may consider an infusion suite to be an important part of your program.

We have discussed time and again that a common growth-limiting resource in an HF program is physician time. Some programs, though, are limited by their physical plant. If a patient has to go to the first floor of your hospital to register, then go to the third floor for an ECG, the fifth floor to have labs drawn, and then come to see you on the second floor, there is ample opportunity for patient flow to be disrupted. The physical layout of your program needs to be patient-friendly and should lend itself to cost-efficient care.

The heart failure clinic

Of course, the HF clinic will require the front-office and back-office functions of any office. For this discussion, I will assume that your HF clinic exists within a practice or hospital that provides those functions. I will focus here on the medical service facilities of your HF clinic. In the HF clinic, your medical director will see patients. In the programs I have developed, as I discussed in the last chapter that there is a close relationship between the medical director and staff in seeing patients. Generally, the nurse case manager or clinical director sees patients with me, so treatment strategies initiated during the visit will be executed smoothly. For example, if I begin spironolactone in a patient, the staff initiates our protocol to monitor potassium levels. If I begin a β-blocker, different protocols are generated. I require a minimum of two exam rooms in the clinic then, so that the details of the therapeutic plan I have begun can be implemented while I move on to the next patient.

We have also discussed how the staff sees patients more frequently than I do. These frequent visits will require two additional exam rooms so as not to interfere with my own efficiency. Four exam rooms, then, will optimize the use of resources for the program for patient flow. Your own needs for a physical facility will depend on your own style of care.

How many exam rooms do you need? One simple approach is to find out the number of patients that came to your practice in the last year with HF CPT codes and the number of office visits these patients represent. If you assume that your program will grow by 25%, and if your program is like others that intensify the number of patient contacts by threefold, you can calculate the number of office hours that your program will generate over the next year (based upon the number of patients that you want to see per hour). This helps you determine the number of exam rooms your program will need. Two rooms 2 days a week would accommodate the needs of the practice in this example:

Number of HF visits in the last year	900	
Projected increase in intensity of outpatient visits	3	$3 \times 900 = 2700$ visits
Projected growth of HF patient population	25%	$2700 \times 1.25 = 3375$ visits
Flow of patients in your practice	3/h	$3375/3 = 1125$ h of visits
Number of office hours/exam room/day in your practice	6	$1125/6 = 187$ days of exam room time
Number of clinic days	2 days/wk $\times$ 50 wk $=$ 100 clinic days	
Number of exam rooms needed for a 2 day/wk HF clinic	$187/100 = 1.87$ exam rooms	

The infusion suite

Infusion therapy can be useful in keeping the sickest patients in your program out of the hospital. An infusion suite can become the focal point of the activity of your program. It is a place to do drug titration visits with fragile patients, a place to administer intravenous diuretics to patients slipping out of control, and a place to administer outpatient infusions of inotropic therapy or B-natriuretic peptide therapy—if you find a role for such treatment in your practice. While scheduled infusion services are no longer mainstream therapy, many programs still use infusions when advanced HF decompensate.

The physical facility used for infusion suites I have visited around the country have ranged from a 6 × 12-ft "closet" to a cavernous 20 × 30-ft suite. The first program I began included telemetry for six infusion patients. Four infusion patients used reclining chairs in the suite. Two chairs for very high risk patients were less comfortable, but allowed cardiopulmonary resuscitation to be done in the chair if necessary. Happily, CPR has never been an issue in my infusion suites, but of course, all supplies needed for emergency intervention need to be available in your program. As a rule of thumb, you should allow 90 ft^2/infusion chair, although my first suite worked with 63 ft^2/infusion chair.

The infusion suite is a patient treatment area that requires a medically sealed, tiled floor. There needs to be a sink and a means to dispose of blood products, sharps, i.v. tubing, etc. There are specific OSHA requirements that must be met. With the administration of i.v. diuretics, natriuretics, aquaretics, and inotropes, easy access to a bathroom is a must.

Building and maintaining an infusion suite entails some work, but this facility can be critical if your goal is a dramatic reduction in HF hospitalizations. It is clearly a setting in which your staff will have frequent contact with your most ill patients. Combined with appropriate therapy, these frequent patient contacts have been shown time and time again to reduce HF hospitalizations and improve quality of life. There is certainly less need to infuse HF patients today, but for a small number of patients, this can still be helpful.

The telemanagement area

This space need not be physically large, but does need to provide patient confidentiality. Patients in an HF program grow very close, but that does not obviate the need for confidentiality. The telephone management area needs to be quiet enough that case managers (or whatever staff is making phone contact in your program) can comfortably discuss private issues with patients. HF affects all aspects of a patient's life. Patient issues and patient management should not be discussed in a public forum.

Support space

As mentioned above, I will assume for this discussion that front-office and back-office space is already being provided within your practice. The additional space needed is office space for the medical and clinical directors and a staff-meeting space. The directors' offices will likely be sized in accordance with your practice norms. The staff-meeting space could be the same as the group education space. If this is not feasible, the staff-meeting space is still important to include in your planning. I like to meet weekly with my staff to review patients and discuss program issues. When planning space, staff space is often the most neglected. This is a mistake in disease management programs that ask more of staff in the delivery of clinical care. The surroundings need not be luxurious, but they need to be adequate to the task. Support space will also include storage areas for the medical supplies needed for the HF clinic and infusion suite, and office supplies.

Summary

A 1500-ft^2 office could easily accommodate the physical plant requirements of your program. These needs include group meeting/education areas, exam rooms of the HF clinic, an infusion suite, a telemanagement office, front- and back-office areas, storage areas, and management office space. If your program is being created within a preexisting practice, many of these areas would be shared with other parts of the practice, making the specific needs of the HF program even more modest. Appropriate accommodation needs to be made, though, for all the activities of the program.

SECTION III

Day-to-day operations

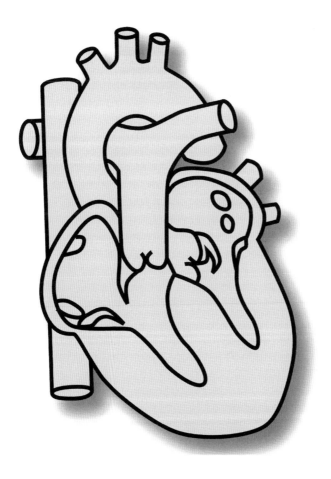

CHAPTER 10

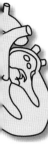

Baseline assessments

Of course you will obtain a baseline history and physical on patients entering your program. National heart failure guidelines also suggest one approach to the initial laboratory evaluation. Your baseline assessment should be careful to include those benchmarks you will use to measure the success of your program. You will also introduce the new patient to your program, begin the patient education program, initiate support from the ancillary personnel, and orient the patient to the resources your program has to offer.

You have built and staffed your facility. You have defined the scope of your program. Financial projections say things are a go. What do you do when that first patient arrives?

The preconsult visit

I have discussed a number of times how I use a preconsult visit to initiate new referrals into our program. This visit makes clear to new patients that they are in a program of HF care, not simply in the care of a physician with an interest in HF. As discussed, we use this opportunity to initiate patient education and to make our baseline assessments.

Quality-of-life assessments

One helpful piece of historical information to collect as a benchmark is an assessment of your patient's functional status. You can certainly design your own quality-of-life (QOL) questionnaire. You could ask, for example, how far a patient can walk before the onset of dyspnea, whether a patient has had to sleep in a chair. You should include your patient's New York Heart Association (NYHA) class in the baseline history and physical as a minimum. There are a number of standardized and validated QOL tools that you can use as well. Some are general assessments of patient QOL and satisfaction, for example the various "short forms" such as SF26. These are not specific to HF, but are widely used.

NYHA functional classes	
Class I	Asymptomatic
Class II	Symptomatic with extraordinary activity
Class IIIA	Symptomatic with ordinary activity
Class IIIB	Symptomatic with minimal activity
Class IV	Symptomatic at rest

There are two standardized QOL questionnaires used in HF clinical trials. The first is the Minnesota Living With Heart Failure Questionnaire.

Minnesota Living With Heart Failure Questionnaire

Did your heart failure prevent you from living as you wanted during the past month by:

	No	Very Little			Very Much
1. Causing swelling in your ankles, legs, etc.?	1	2	3	4	5
2. Making your working around the house or yard difficult?	1	2	3	4	5
3. Making your relating to or doing things with your friends or family difficult?	1	2	3	4	5
4. Making you sit or lie down to rest during the day?	1	2	3	4	5
5. Making you tired, fatigued or low on energy?	1	2	3	4	5
6. Making your working to earn a living difficult?	1	2	3	4	5
7. Making your walking about or climbing stairs difficult?	1	2	3	4	5
8. Making you short of breath?	1	2	3	4	5
9. Making your sleeping at night difficult?	1	2	3	4	5
10. Making you eat less of the foods you like?	1	2	3	4	5
11. Making your going places away from home difficult?	1	2	3	4	5
12. Making your sexual activities difficult?	1	2	3	4	5
13. Making your recreational pastimes, sports or hobbies difficult?	1	2	3	4	5

14. Making it difficult for you to concentrate and remember things?	1	2	3	4	5
15. Giving you side effects from medicines?	1	2	3	4	5
16. Making you worry?	1	2	3	4	5
17. Making you feel depressed?	1	2	3	4	5
18. Costing you money for medical care?	1	2	3	4	5
19. Making you feel a loss of self control of your life?	1	2	3	4	5
20. Making you stay in a hospital?	1	2	3	4	5
21. Making you feel you are a burden to your family or friends?	1	2	3	4	5

You will need to obtain permission if you are going to use this tool in your HF program. There are other QOL instruments available as well, such as the Kansas City Cardiomyopathy score. These also require permission for you to use in your program.

The Kansas City Cardiomyopathy Questionnaire

The following questions refer to your heart failure and how it may affect your life. Please read and complete the following questions. There are no right or wrong answers. Please mark the answer that best applies to you.

1 Heart failure affects different people in different ways. Some feel shortness of breath while others feel fatigue. Please indicate how much you are limited by heart failure (shortness of breath or fatigue) in your ability to do the following activities over the past 2 weeks.

Activity	Extremely limited	Quite a bit limited	Moderately limited	Slightly limited	Not at all limited	Limited for other reasons or did not do the activity
Dressing yourself	o	o	o	o	o	o
Showering/bathing	o	o	o	o	o	o
Walking 1 block on level ground	o	o	o	o	o	o
Doing yard work, housework or carrying groceries	o	o	o	o	o	o
Climbing a flight of stairs without stopping	o	o	o	o	o	o
Hurrying or jogging (as if to catch a bus)	o	o	o	o	o	o

2 Compared with 2 weeks ago, have your symptoms of heart failure (shortness of breath, fatigue, or ankle swelling) changed? My symptoms of heart failure have become . . .

Much worse	Slightly worse	Not changed	Slightly better	Much better	I've had no symptoms over the last 2 weeks
o	o	o	o	o	o

3 Over the past 2 weeks, how many times did you have swelling in your feet, ankles or legs when you woke up in the morning?

Every morning	3 or more times a week, but not every day	1–2 times a week	Less than once a week	Never over the past 2 weeks
o	o	o	o	o

4 Over the past 2 weeks, how much has swelling in your feet, ankles or legs bothered you?

Extremely bothersome	Quite a bit bothersome	Moderately bothersome	Slightly bothersome	Not at all bothersome	I've had no swelling
o	o	o	o	o	o

5 Over the past 2 weeks, on average, how many times has fatigue limited your ability to do what you want?

All of the time	Several times per day	At least once a day	3 or more times per week but not not every day	1–2 times per week	Less than once a week	Never over the past 2 weeks
o	o	o	o	o	o	o

6 Over the past 2 weeks, how much has your fatigue bothered you?

Extremely bothersome	Quite a bit bothersome	Moderately bothersome	Slightly bothersome	Not at all bothersome	I've had no fatigue
o	o	o	o	o	o

7 Over the past 2 weeks, on average, how many times has shortness of breath limited you ability to do what you wanted?

All of the time	Several times per day	At least once a day	3 or more times per week but not every day	1–2 times per week	Less than once a week	Never over the past 2 weeks
o	o	o	o	o	o	o

8 Over the past 2 weeks, how much has your shortness of breath bothered you?

Extremely bothersome	Quite a bit bothersome	Moderately bothersome	Slightly bothersome	Not at all bothersome	I've had no shortness of breath
o	o	o	o	o	o

9 Over the past 2 weeks, on average, how many times have you been forced to sleep sitting up in a chair or with at least 3 pillows to prop you up because of shortness of breath.

Every night	3 or more times a week, but not every day	1–2 times a week	Less than once a week	Never over the the past 2 weeks
o	o	o	o	o

10 Heart failure symptoms can worsen for a number of reasons. How sure are you that you know what to do, or whom to call, if your heart failure gets worse?

Not at all sure	Not very sure	Somewhat sure	Mostly sure	Completely sure
o	o	o	o	o

11 How well do you understand what things you are able to do to keep your heart failure symptoms from getting worse? (for example, weighing yourself, eating a low salt diet, etc.)

Do not understand at all	Do not understand very well	Somewhat understand	Mostly understand	Completely understand
o	o	o	o	o

12 Over the past 2 weeks, how much has your heart failure limited your enjoyment of life?

It has extremely limited my enjoyment of life	It has limited my enjoyment of life quite a bit	It has moderately limited my enjoyment of life	It has slightly limited my enjoyment of life	It has not limited my enjoyment of life at all
o	o	o	o	o

13 If you had to spend the rest of your life with your heart failure the way it is right now, how would you feel about this?

Not at all satisfied	Mostly dissatisfied	Somewhat satisfied	Mostly satisfied	Completely satisfied
o	o	o	o	o

14 Over the past 2 weeks, how often have you felt discouraged or down in the dumps because of your heart failure?

I felt that way all of the time	I felt that way most of the time	I occasionally felt that way	I rarely felt that way	I never felt that way
o	o	o	o	o

15 How much does your heart failure affect your lifestyle? Please indicate how your heart failure may have limited your participation in the following activities over the past 2 weeks.

Activity	Severely limited	Limited quite a bit	Moderately limited	Slightly limited	Did not limit at all	Does not apply or did not do for other reasons
Hobbies, recreational activities	o	o	o	o	o	o
Working or doing household chores	o	o	o	o	o	o
Visiting family or friends out of your home	o	o	o	o	o	o
Intimate relationships with loved ones	o	o	o	o	o	o

I also have the staff administer a questionnaire to establish the patient's level of understanding of HF and its treatment. Unfortunately, patients commonly have little idea of what HF is, how it developed, and what their prognosis is. Often, the terms "heart failure" and "heart attack" are confused by patients.

As sleep apnea is so common in HF patients, an assessment of sleep is an appropriate part of the baseline assessment. There are two widely used tools for this: the Berlin and Epworth questionnaires. Each has proponents and detractors, so I use both. The Epworth Questionnaire is most widely used by sleep laboratories.

Berlin Questionnaire

CATEGORY ONE:
1. Do you snore?
2. How loud is your snoring?
   As loud as breathing
   As loud as talking

Louder than talking

Loud enough to be heard in the next room

3. How often do you snore?

Nearly every day

3–4 × / week

1–2 × / week

1–2 × / month

Hardly ever

4. Has your snoring ever bothered other people?

5. Has anyone noticed you stop breathing when you are asleep?

Nearly every day

3–4 × / week

1–2 × / week

1–2 × / month

Hardly ever

Category I is positive if any of the above is present.

CATEGORY TWO:

1. After sleep, are you fatigued?

3–4 × / week

1–2 × / week

1–2 × / month

Hardly ever

2. While awake, are you fatigued?

3–4 × / week

1–2 × / week

1–2 × / month

Hardly ever

3. Have you ever fallen asleep while driving a vehicle?

Nearly every day

3–4 × / week

1–2 × / week

1–2 × / month

Hardly ever

Category II is positive if any of the above is present.

CATEGORY THREE:

1. Do you have hypertension?

2. Is your BMI >30?

Category III is positive if any of the above is present.

You are at high risk for sleep disorder if two or more categories are positive.

Epworth Sleepiness Scale

How likely are you to doze off or fall asleep in the following situations?
(in contrast to just feeling tired) Use the following scale to rate your chance
of dozing in the following situations:

Situation	Chance of Dozing
(refers to your usual way of life in recent times. Even if you have not done some of these things recently, try to work out how they would have affected you).	• 0 = would never doze • 1 = slight chance of dozing • 2 = moderate chance of dozing • 3 = high chance of dozing

Sitting and reading
Watching TV
Sitting, inactive, in a public place
As a passenger in a car for an hour
Lying down in the afternoon
Sitting and talking to someone
Sitting quietly after a lunch without alcohol

TOTAL

Score Analysis

• Score of 1–6: you're getting enough sleep
• Score of 4–8: you tend to be sleepy during the day; this is the average score
• Score of 9–15: you are very sleepy and should seek medical advice
• **Score of 16 or greater:** you are dangerously sleepy and should seek medical advice

Because of the interaction between HF therapies such as β-blockers and aldosterone antagonists and sexual function, I also take advantage of the preconsult visit to obtain a baseline assessment of erectile dysfunction (ED). We use this simple tool:

Sexual Health Inventory for Men Questionnaire

This questionnaire is designed to help you and your doctor determine if you may be experiencing ED. Knowing everything you can about ED means you're better prepared to make the most important step of all: getting treatment.

Each question has several possible responses. Choose the one that best describes your own situation. Your results are private. Only you will see them.

Over the past 6 months:

1. How would you rate your confidence in your ability to get and keep an erection?

   ☐ Very Low
   ☐ Low
   ☐ Moderate
   ☐ High
   ☐ Very High

2. When you had erections with sexual stimulation, how often were your erections hard enough for penetration (entering your partner)?

   ☐ No sexual activity
   ☐ Almost never/never
   ☐ A few times (much less than half the time)
   ☐ Sometimes (about half the time)
   ☐ Most times (much more than half the time)
   ☐ Almost always/always

3. During sexual intercourse, how often were you able to maintain your erection after you had penetrated (entered) your partner?

   ☐ Did not attempt intercourse
   ☐ Almost never/never
   ☐ A few times (much less than half the time)
   ☐ Sometimes (about half the time)
   ☐ Most times (much more than half the time)
   ☐ Almost always/always

4. During sexual intercourse, how difficult was it to maintain your erection to completion of intercourse?

   ☐ Did not attempt intercourse
   ☐ Extremely difficult

□ Very difficult
□ Difficult
□ Slightly difficult
□ Not difficult

5. When you attempted sexual intercourse, how often was it satisfactory for you?

□ Did not attempt intercourse
□ Almost never/never
□ A few times (much less than half the time)
□ Sometimes (about half the time)
□ Most times (much more than half the time)
□ Almost always/always

Diagnostic testing

I have already listed the other measurements that I use in the preconsult visit to assess the HF status of patients entering the program. In addition to assuring that there is a recent ECG and echocardiogram on file, I ask my staff to do a 6-minute walk with patients, as well as a noninvasive measurement of hemodynamics with the Cardiodynamics Bio-Z. Laboratory parameters include a B-natriuretic peptide measurement and a platelet function assay for aspirin resistance. Home testing for sleep apnea is also appropriate for new patients.

The initial consult

Of course you will get a medical history and physical (H&P) examination on each patient. Accepting an H&P from outside your program is a mistake. It is unusual for such an outside H&P to reveal the etiology of a patient's HF, the details of prior exercise tests, catheterizations, intracoronary interventions, and bypass surgeries. Commonly, the left ventricular ejection fraction (LVEF) will not be recorded. The reason an angiotensin receptor blocker (ARB) is being used rather than an angiotensin-converting enzyme (ACE) inhibitor is rarely noted. Patient information is usually scattered between office and hospital charts. You need to have all of this information before you can formulate your treatment goals and strategies. Documentation here is very important, especially if several of the next few visits to your HF program will be "incident to" visits.

Noninvasive Hemodynamic Assessment (Bio-Z)

Parameter	Description	Value	Low	Normal	High
HR	Heart rate	89	58	86	
SBP	Systolic blood pressure	104	100	140	
DBP	Diastolic blood pressure	58	40	90	
MAP	Mean arterial pressure	71	84	100	
CI	Cardiac index	1.9	2.5	4.7	
CO	Cardiac output	2.9	3.9	7.3	
SI	Stroke index	21	35	65	
SV	Stroke volume	32	54	101	
SVRI	Systemic vascular Res. index	2770	1337	2483	
SVR	Systemic vascular resistance	1798	742	1378	
ACI	Acceleration index	72	90	170	
VI	Velocity index	24	33	65	
TFC	Thoracic fluid content	33.0	21.0	37.0	
LCWI	Left cardiac work index	1.6	3.0	5.5	
LCW	Left cardiac work	2.5	5.4	10.0	
STR	Systolic time ratio	0.56	0.30	0.50	
PEP	Preejection period	131			
LVET	Left ventricular ejection Time	232			

There is another reason to get your own detailed H&P. Like all physicians, you want to know where a patient has been and where they are today so you can plot the future course you will pursue. Unlike other physicians, you will need to prove to payors and your colleagues that your program works, so you will have to make a patient's baseline status absolutely clear upon entering the program so that it can be reviewed later by a third party. Unless you can prove that you have increased the use of ACE inhibitors from 50 to 91% in your patients, no one will believe you. Part of your H&P, then, will be to include such information. No one counts the number of HF hospitalizations a patient has had in the last year. If you do not record this in your H&P, this will be very difficult information to get later, and thus it will be very difficult to prove that you decreased hospitalization rates in your patients, a key goal of disease management programs. If the patient has not had a recent LVEF measurement upon entry into your program, how will you show your intensive program of education and monitoring made a difference? To capture the specific information that you want on every new patient, you might want to consider a baseline form containing patient demographics and any variables you want to use to create benchmarks for measuring clinical outcomes.

Laboratory assessments

In addition to the H&P, each patient entering an HF program will need certain baseline laboratory measurements. These include a comprehensive metabolic profile to check electrolytes, liver function, and renal function. Calcium and magnesium levels are also important. Thyroid-stimulating hormone levels will identify hypothyroidism as a secondary cause of HF in several patients each year in a typical HF program. The current guidelines also recommend a CBC, ferritin, and transferrin saturation. Obtaining a B-natriuretic peptide level is growing in importance as part of a baseline evaluation.

While a urinalysis is part of the standard evaluation, urinary cate-cholamines and screening for connective tissue disease is now considered optional testing. A chest X-ray and electrocardiogram should be obtained on each patient. While viral titers for agents such as CMV are no longer recommended as they are rarely helpful in determining the course of therapy, HIV testing is now encouraged.

Choosing your benchmarks

Your baseline assessments have two purposes. First, it is important to clearly identify the etiology of HF in each patient. Secondly, these measurements will be used to monitor progress over time. These measurements will form part of the benchmarks for your programs outcome measurements. Before you do your H&P, you need to decide what outcomes you want to measure. You also need to decide on the benchmarks by which you want your program to be judged. Do you want to use your patients as their own control? For example, will you be comparing hospitalization rates in the year before program entry to the hospitalization rates of your patients in the year after entering your program? Or do you want to compare your patients to the regional or national hospitalization rates you can obtain from Medicare? Do you want to compare the HF patients in your practice who are in your program to HF patients in your practice that your partners did not refer to you? Or should you compare the HF patients in your program to HF patients of an insurance carrier with whom you are trying to get a contract? Whatever data you gather, you will probably be ahead of your competitors. You will do yourself a great favor, though, by giving considerable thought to what you want to measure as you set up your protocols.

You would be wise to choose benchmarks that will clearly reflect the success of your program. If you choose the wrong benchmarks, a successful

HF program might actually demonstrate an unintended adverse impact on that outcome. For example, you might think that a good benchmark is the length of stay (LOS) of those HF patients from your program who are hospitalized. However, you might be surprised to learn that LOS could actually increase. The short "tune up" admissions are gone. Once you are running a successful HF program, the only patients who are now admitted are the profoundly ill patients who cannot be handled in your infusion suite or with intense telemanagement. HF patients admitted from a top notch HF program are the sorts of patients that often need intubation or who require intra-aortic balloon pump support. LOS for these sick patients is longer than for most HF patients.

Likewise, total hospitalizations can go up if your program is working well, as your HF patients now feel well enough for that carpal tunnel surgery or cataract surgery. Proclaiming that your program has doubled the LOS for the HF DRG 127 or that you have increased total hospitalizations by 50% may not impress your hospital administrator or the insurance payor.

There are benchmarks that you can affect. You may do better to choose the number of HF hospitalizations as your benchmark rather than LOS. This is an outcome that will reflect the success of your program. If you are doing a good job, fewer patients should decompensate to the point of requiring hospitalization. If you do not choose your benchmarks, someone else may choose them for you. It is clearly worth the effort to collect your own data and choose your own endpoints.

Layering outcomes

It is important to show that you are successful as early as possible. Some outcomes, such as the number of HF hospitalizations, take time to gather. You can measure your early success by layering outcomes, i.e., gathering some short-term, some intermediate-term, and some long-term outcomes. By layering outcomes, an HF program can demonstrate early results, and then follow up with continually more sophisticated data. For example, a short-term outcome may be measuring the percentage of patients on ACE inhibitors, β-blockers, and spironolactone. By 6 months, measurements of QOL, NYHA class, LVEF, B-natriuretic peptide levels, and 6-minute-walk distance can give intermediate-term outcomes. Long-term hospitalization rates and mortality can be assessed to determine your program's effect on these parameters. I suggest obtaining benchmark data at 0, 3, 6, and 12 months, and then yearly thereafter.

Layering outcomes

Short-term:
• Optimization of medications
• Noninvasive hemodynamic measurements
• B-natriuretic peptides
Intermediate-term:
• QOL questionnaires
• Educational assessments of HF knowledge
• NYHA class
• LVEF
• 6-min-walk test
• Cardiopulmonary stress testing
• Noninvasive hemodynamic measurements
• B-natriuretic peptides
Long-term:
• HF hospitalizations
• Mortality
• Serial measurements of intermediate outcomes

The treatment plan

Once you have your own H&P in hand, a QOL measurement, functional assessments, and nutritional assessments, and have collected the outcome markers by which you will assess your program's success, your patient is ready to enter the treatment phase of your program. You should now have a good idea of the etiology, history, and tempo of your patient's heart failure.

The next step is to set up goals and a treatment plan for the patient. These goals should be simple, practical, and taken one at a time. My short-term goals may be to optimize a patient's ACE inhibitors, β-blockers, and spironolactone. I may need a cardiac catheterization to complete my database. I will start the education process to teach the patient and family about HF and its treatment. I will need to fill in any gaps in the initial database, looking in particular for any reversible etiologies of HF such as hypothyroidism or treatable etiologies such as mitral regurgitation.

I also ask the patient to articulate his or her own short-, medium-, and long-range goals. These are recorded, so we can keep the patient's needs in mind as well. Recording these goals also helps when explaining to a patient who is complaining that he can only work as a security guard for 6 hours a day that his original goal was to be able to take the trash to the curb without dyspnea. Creating a formal treatment plan gets you, your HF staff, your patient, and the patient's family on the same page. The establishment of short- and long-term goals emphasizes to everyone that we have engaged in a lifelong process. Your benchmark measurements will then tell you if you are on track with your treatment plan.

Summary

The baseline assessment of your new patient is the foundation of the care you will provide for your patient for some time. Your baseline assessment will convince the patient that you and your staff are expert in HF care, which should lead to more compliance. It will establish the etiology and status of your patient's HF, which will illuminate the treatment path and lead to better patient outcomes. Further, collecting this information at the outset will allow you to prove to others that your program is providing good care.

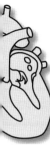

CHAPTER 11

Heart failure clinic follow-up visits

Day-to-day patient care focuses on educating, educating, and reeducating the patient and then intensively monitoring patient progress to make therapy proactive rather than reactive. Telemanagement is crucial to the monitoring effort. To speed clinical decision making, therapeutic algorithms can be protocol driven to allow your staff to perform ongoing titration of therapy.

During your baseline assessment, your goal was to determine where your patient was in the spectrum of the HF disease process, how he or she got there, and where you want to take him or her in the future. You also did baseline testing, so you could measure her progress by the benchmarks you have chosen. Now we turn to the process of achieving the clinical outcomes implied by those benchmarks. You are not the only one setting standards for your HF care. The ACC/AHA performance standards for your clinic visits are already in place. There are a number of parameters that are expected to be memorialized in the medical record. The performance measure is determined by the percentage of visits in which the performance measures are met:

ACC/AHA Performance Measures

History
Symptoms of volume overload recorded / # visits
Activity level assessed / # visits
      (NYHA/MLWHFQ/KCCQ/CHFQ [Guyatt])

Physical
Signs of volume overload recorded / # visits
Heart exam / # visits

Lab
Initial CBC, BMP, Ca^{2+}, Mg^{2+}, LFTs, TSH
Serial electrolytes and renal function
Weight measurement / # visits
BP measurement / # visits

Patient education documented q6 months
β-blocker given for systolic dysfunction
ACE inhibitor given for systolic dysfunction
Warfarin given for atrial fibrillation

The ACC/AHA performance measures have been shown not to influence HF hospitalizations. This is not entirely surprising. Starting warfarin for atrial fibrillation is unlikely to affect HF hospitalizations in the short-term, even if it is the right thing to do. To meet the standard for patient education, a number of issues must be specifically addressed according to the ACC/AHA performance measures.

Issues to address in an HF program

Weight monitoring
Diet (sodium restriction)
Symptom management
Physical activity
Smoking cessation
Medication instruction
Minimize/avoid NSAIDs
Follow-up plans
Referral for specific education program
Prognosis/end-of-life issues

These are not the only standards to consider in constructing your HF disease management program. There are other, sometimes competing, standards. We now have national guidelines that also delineate what kinds of education a disease management program should provide. The Heart Failure Society of America (HFSA) guidelines are most specific as to the kinds of patient education that are worthy of receiving their highest level of recommendation:

8.1 It is recommended that patients with HF and their family members or caregivers receive individualized education and counseling that emphasizes self-care. This education and counseling should be delivered by providers using a team approach in which nurses with expertise in HF management provide the majority of education and counseling, supplemented by physician input and, when available and needed, input from dieticians, pharmacists, and other health care providers. All HF patients benefit from education and counseling, but patients in NYHA functional class III or IV need the most intensive education, while patients in NYHA I or II need less intensive education.

Teaching is not sufficient without skill building and specification of critical target behaviors.

The HFSA guidelines go on to define the "essential elements of patient education..."

Essential elements of patient education

Definition of HF (linking disease, symptoms, and treatment) and the cause of patient's HF

Recognition of escalating symptoms and selection of appropriate treatments in response to particular symptoms

Indications and use of each medicine

Importance of risk factor modification

Therapeutic lifestyle dietary modifications

Therapeutic lifestyle exercise modifications

Strategies to improve compliance

Your program would do well to consider this advice in constructing the educational component of your program. While education is traditionally a poorly reimbursed activity, it is clearly in the patients' interests to educate, educate, and reeducate HF patients in the sorts of behaviors that will minimize their hospitalizations and rehospitalizations.

An educational questionnaire I have given to assess patients at baseline and every 6 months is this:

Educational Questionnaire

How did you develop HF?
What are the signs of HF?
What are the symptoms of HF?
Are you taking an ACE inhibitor?
What is its name?
What is its dose?
Are you taking a β-blocker?
What is its name?
What is its dose?
What is your daily fluid budget?
What is your daily sodium budget?

What is your dry weight?
Which of your medicines make you breathe easier?
Which of your medicines make you live longer?
Which of your medicines affect your potassium levels?

It is likely that patients entering your program will be able to answer few, if any, of these questions. After you have optimized the medical regimen the patients should be able to do well on this questionnaire. If not, you may need to reassess your educational effort.

Group visits

Treatment goals can be met through individual and group visits. After the initial consult, we offer patients the option of receiving their care through individual or group visits. I have been surprised at the popularity of group visits. In a previous chapter, I introduced the concept of the CHCC (Community Health Continuity Clinic) group visits for continuity of care and the DIGMA (drop-in group medical appointment) model for episodic problems. Both types of group visits require a HIPPA waiver. Care will be delivered, after all, in a group setting, so privacy issues are involved.
Again referring to the HFSA guidelines:

> 8.3 It is recommended that educational sessions begin with an assessment of current HF knowledge, issues about which the patient wants to learn, and the patient's perceived barriers to change. Address specific issues (e.g. medication nonadherence) and their causes (e.g. lack of knowledge vs cost vs forgetting) and employ strategies that promote behavior change, including motivational approaches.

Group visits must involve the delivery of patient care. They are interactive, but they are not a support group and are not for educational purposes only. In the CHCC model, 20 patients are seen for 90 minutes. A prescribing healthcare professional and a nurse run the group.
The first 10-minute portion of the meeting is for reminiscence. The group discusses their HF, establishing the commonality of the patients in that they all have HF. Next, the core curriculum is addressed. In my programs, a series of four CHCC group visits are offered:

Group visits

Visit I: The causes, signs, and symptoms of HF.
Therapeutic lifestyle changes (fluid and sodium budgets, weight monitoring)
Diuretic therapy

Visit II: Testing of information covered in visit I.
The "live longer" vs. "feel better" medications of HF
Drug–drug interactions

Visit III: Testing of information covered in visit II.
The self-management of HF.
Dealing with hyperkalemia, hypokalemia, and hypotension

Visit IV: Testing of information covered in visit III.
The testing is used to monitor HF

Next, there is a working break, during which the nurse gets vital signs and the prescribing healthcare professional addresses the patient problems one at a time. This is followed by a Q&A session and a discussion about what will be covered at the next session. Finally, one-on-one time is offered to the patients in the group.

The fear of most physicians is that in offering one-on-one time, all of the patients in the group will choose that option. Nationally, on average only about a quarter of patients ask for additional private sessions following the group meetings. In my experience, the proportion is much less than that.

CHCC visits do work, reducing HF hospitalizations 12% and emergency department visits 18%. Your task is not done at the end of this series of four visits, of course. The series is, nonetheless, a good start. After all, $7 \times 1 = 0$, while $3 \times 3 = 2$. Patient education is a relentless goal for an HF program.

Therapeutic goals in the clinic

During the first visit, patients in my program receive an orientation packet containing the phone numbers, pager numbers, and on-call numbers to use to contact the HF staff. We then teach the patients when to call us. HF patients are resource intensive, needy patients with a chronic, incurable disease. We want our patients to call when they are confused or in trouble. On the other hand, we do not want to be overwhelmed with unnecessary phone calls. Still, the strength of a disease management program is a proactive, aggressive care strategy based on early recognition of symptoms and early intervention before things have progressed to the point of hospitalization.

HF treatment is a long-term proposition. Like any relationship, we have to get used to the individual needs of each patient, and they need to

get used to our program. Over time, it is not difficult to train patients
when to call and when not to call. This training is an early goal of treatment. Each patient is different. Some need more support; others are more
independent.

When to call us

The success we will have fighting your HF will depend on recognizing
your symptoms early and looking for signs that your HF is slipping out
of control. Look for these signs and call XZY HF program when you find
them:
- Increasing fatigue or breathlessness
- Swelling in your ankles and hands
- Bloating of your stomach
- Needing more pillows at night to be comfortable
- Waking up at night short of breath or coughing
- A weight gain of

  2 lb in a night . . .
  5 lb in a week . . .
  5 lb over your dry weight
  (your dry weight is _____ lb)

  Call 911 if you have:
- Worsening chest tightness or chest pain
- A cough with pink frothy sputum

Increasing compliance

There is no question that one of the ways disease management programs
achieve superior clinical outcomes is to improve patient compliance with
standard medical regimens. Cheerleading for chronically ill patients is not
a core skill of many physicians; physician extenders are generally much
better suited for this task. Our simple formula for compliance is to educate, educate, and reeducate patients; and then to monitor, monitor, and
remonitor patients' progress.

   Compliance with a multidrug regimen is not easy. Once a patient is taking more than three medications (as all HF patients do), noncompliance
approaches 50%. If the drugs are costly (as HF drugs are) or have side
effects (as HF drugs do) noncompliance rates are even higher. Patients

are not happy taking drugs for life, especially if their HF symptoms diminish. Noncompliance is a major reason why HF is the leading cause of hospitalization and rehospitalization. I have watched my staff spend hours with some patients reviewing and re-reviewing medications over multiple clinic visits and phone calls. This requires incredible patience—more than I have quite frankly. I'm glad my staff embraces the task.

To improve compliance, we intensely educate our patients about the signs and symptoms of HF. We discuss treatments that will help patients feel better (inotropes, diuretics) and those that prolong life (ACE Is/ARBs, β-blockers, spironolactone, hydralazine/nitrates). If the patients understand how congestive symptoms occur, it is a little less likely they will mistakenly overload themselves with salt and fluid. Without education, I have had numerous HF patients force fluids while they are on diuretics "to replace what I pee'd out." Education cannot be replaced as a central component of HF therapy.

We repeatedly go over medications, what they do, and what side effects to expect. I think the educational questionnaire helps, too. A patient who can name his or her medications and the rationale behind their use is less likely to skip doses. Through careful monitoring and telemanagement, it is less likely a patient will run out of his or her medicines while on vacation.

Simply asking at each visit in a nonjudgmental way about compliance has uncovered many problems with which we can help. Taking bid diuretics can cause nocturia, so moving up the second dose to noon can eliminate that problem. Adjusting the timing of ACEI and β-blockers can avoid fatigue and dizziness. Medicines are more likely to be taken if the regimen fits in with a patient's daily routine.

We give each patient a fresh list of the medications with each visit. This forces a discussion; often we will change to once daily dosing or simplify the regimen in some other way if compliance problems crop up. Giving pillboxes or other reminder systems, such as refrigerator magnets, has been helpful. Enlisting spouses, friends, and family can be important if a patient's memory is not the best.

The patients have to assume responsibility for their own health. I can help by assisting the patients in understanding their disease. Often I have to clarify what a patient has heard from friends, seen on television, or read in the newspaper.

Again, the most successful strategy we have found is to educate, educate, and reeducate; and then to monitor, monitor, and remonitor results. An open dialogue about compliance, especially with physician extenders in your program, is important to achieve the outcomes you want.

Risk factors for noncompliance

- Inability to get along with your HF staff and a high level of anger chronically
- Multiple missed and rescheduled clinic visits
- A pattern of nonreturned phone calls and general inaccessibility
- Inability to list medications and dosing frequency
- Lack of achievement of education milestones (e.g., knowing daily fluid and sodium budgets or target dry weight)
- Complaints about lack of clinical improvement, cost of therapy, and/or side effects
- Denial of severity of disease, rationalizing signs, and symptoms
- Taking more than three different medications

Implementing therapeutic lifestyle changes

Getting patients to recognize the importance of dietary support is difficult. The advice of a dietician is dreaded because it is assumed the advice will mean deprivation of the simple joys in life. Still I have had a considerable number of patients where dietary support made all the difference. We often include dietary visits with nursing staff visits. This justifies the complexity of the "incident to" billing submitted for services that day and decreases the "no show" visits we saw when dietary visits were on a separate day.

Tools for helping patients with daily fluid budgets

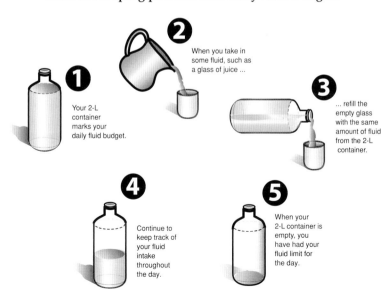

1 Your 2-L container marks your daily fluid budget.

2 When you take in some fluid, such as a glass of juice ...

3 ... refill the empty glass with the same amount of fluid from the 2-L container.

4 Continue to keep track of your fluid intake throughout the day.

5 When your 2-L container is empty, you have had your fluid limit for the day.

All of our staff, and especially our dietician, stress sodium and fluid budgets at every visit. Along with monitoring of daily weight, these budgets are the most important parameters to follow in tracking therapeutic lifestyle changes in HF. Practical physical examples help bring compliance home. If I tell a patient that they have a 2-L fluid budget, their first question is usually "What is a liter?" Converting to the English system of measurement helps. Patients can relate to eight cups of fluid a day and can understand that anything that wiggles, jiggles, or melts at room temperature is a fluid. We tell patients to use a 2-L soda bottle to track their fluid budget each day.

Monitoring dietary sodium is more elusive than monitoring fluid intake and body weight. The creativity of our dietician in getting this information from patients is impressive. Telling a patient to adhere to a 2000 mg sodium budget usually leads to the question "What is a milligram?" Again, physical models and concrete examples can help the patient understand this concept. Since one teaspoon of salt contains 2100 mg of sodium, removing the saltshaker from the table and cutting the salt in recipes in half is a practical first step in budgeting. Learning to read food labels and limiting sodium to 600 mg/meal is also important.

Most Americans are overweight or obese. In patients with heart disease, this is especially problematic. Nutritional support for these obese HF patients with the reasonable and achievable goal of a 10% loss of body weight (as opposed to trying to achieve ideal body weight) can have substantial impact. We use a number of tools to assess our patients' nutritional status at the initial visit and at subsequent benchmark visits.

Nutritional Assessment Form

Name _____

1. Are you currently following a specific diet?
   ☐ Yes ☐ No
   If yes, what type of diet?_____

2. Have you previously been instructed on a low-sodium diet?
   ☐ Yes ☐ No
   If yes, when and by whom? _____

3. Do you add salt to your foods?
   ☐ Yes ☐ No

4. Do you use salt in cooking?

   ☐ Yes ☐ No

5. Do you use a salt substitute?

   ☐ Yes ☐ No

   If yes, which one? _____

6. Have you been instructed to limit your fluid intake?

   ☐ Yes ☐ No

   If yes, how much fluid are you allowed per day? _____

7. How much beer, wine, or liquor do you drink per week? _____

8. What beverages do you generally drink?

   ☐ Coffee ☐ Colas ☐ Sports drinks

   ☐ Tea ☐ Diet colas ☐ Fruit juice

   ☐ Water ☐ Milk ☐ Other

9. Who does most of the grocery shopping and food preparation at your home?

   ☐ Self ☐ Spouse ☐ Other

10. How many times per week do you eat at restaurants?

   ☐ Daily

   ☐ 1–2 times per week

   ☐ 3 or more times per week

   ☐ 2–3 times per month

   ☐ Rarely

Dietary Recall Diary

Please list everything you had to eat and drink yesterday. Include water and all beverages. Also include the size of each serving and the way it was prepared.

Food	Amount	Preparation Method

Food Frequency Checklist

Please check how often you consume the following foods:

Food	Daily	1–2 times/week	1–2 times/month	Rarely/never
Canned soup				
Canned vegetables				
Frozen dinners				
Instant potatoes				
Box mixes				
Hot dogs				
Lunch meat				
Sausage				
Cheese				
Salad dressing				
Catsup/mustard				
Soy sauce				
Potato chips				
Pretzels				
Gatorade				
Fast food				

In addition to education, the clinic visits, whether group or individual, spend considerable effort to apply and optimize evidence-based therapy. This starts with applying the national guidelines, but often extends beyond guideline-sanctioned therapy. Guidelines rest on proven therapies. In a chronic, lethal incurable disease such as HF, the role of the clinician is to weigh the available evidence and apply it to individual patients. The inclusion and exclusion criteria of clinical trials on which guidelines are based often define the use of a given therapy only for a narrow patient cohort. Your patients come in all ages, genders, sizes, and shapes. They have a spectrum of comorbidities. The treating clinician has to decide when clinical trial results can be generalized to other patients. We will consider drug titrations in the next chapter.

You will monitor patient progress at every contact, but in particular at benchmark visits. I have found that these benchmark visits need to be scheduled separately, otherwise they never get done. In addition, the benchmark visits tend to be longer visits, so appropriate time needs to be set aside for completing the questionnaires, the 6-minute walk, etc.

Summary

After the initial evaluation, the real work of HF care begins. A major thrust of clinic visits is to educate patients about HF and then monitor their progress. The education can occur in both the individual and group visit setting. The monitoring occurs at these visits as well, but occurs more formally at visits set aside to measure the parameters you have chosen as the benchmarks of your program.

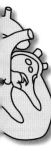

CHAPTER 12

Medical treatment protocols

While each patient is unique, most medication initiation and up- or downtitration can be done by protocol. In our hands, fewer HF patients "fall through the cracks" when receiving protocol-driven therapy than when all therapeutic decisions go through the physician. You should write your own protocols and adapt them to your treatment style. Here I list some protocols that I've seen in various HF programs. You should consider these as a starting point only, without any endorsement as to whether they are appropriate for your situation.

It is beyond the scope of this book to review how HF should be treated. The medical director of your program will decide, for example, when you are going to use ACE inhibitors, when you will use ARBs, and when you will use both. Once you have decided on which therapy to use for a patient, your staff will find it helpful to have formal protocols to use during the "incident to" drug titration visits. For ACE inhibitor therapy, for example, the following protocol could be used:

Protocol ACE inhibitors

1 Choose an ACE inhibitor based upon specific needs of the patient. Once-a-day dosing, low-cost, and good tissue penetration are desirable features. Using an ACE inhibitor at a dose clinically proven to be efficacious in a HF clinical trial is also important.

2 Obtain baseline renal function and serum electrolytes prior to initiating ACE inhibitor. Repeat renal function and chemistry analysis 1 week after an increase in dose, or if symptoms occur. A Bio-Z can also be obtained if there is a question as to whether the patient will tolerate the next dose titration.

3 Start titration at one-fourth to one-half of the target dosage and titrate upward toward maximum dosing weekly/every other week as clinical symptoms, blood pressure, and laboratory results allow. Target doses of ACE inhibitor from HF trials are:

Tissue ACE inhibitors
- Mavik (trandolapril)   4 mg q.d.
- Monopril (fosinopril)   40 mg q.d.
- Altace (ramipril)   5 mg b.i.d.

Nontissue ACE inhibitors
- Vasotec (enalapril)   20 mg b.i.d.
- Zestril/Prinivil (lisinopril) 30–40 mg q.d.
- Capoten (captopril)   50 mg t.i.d.

Titration schedule for ACE inhibitor on formulary

Week	Lisinopril (Prinivil, Zestril) (mg q.d.)	Ramipril (Altace) (mg q.d.)	Enalapril (Vasotec) (mg q.d.)
1	5.0	2.5	2.5
3	10.0	5.0	5.0
5	20.0	7.5	7.5
7	40.0	10.0	10.0

4 Monitor blood pressure and clinical symptoms during titration via clinic visits or telemanagement. Do not uptitrate unless BP is stable and is >90 mm Hg systolic.

5 Evaluate electrolyte and blood urea nitrogen/creatinine levels during the titration phase:

a If the creatinine level rises 0.5 mg/dL, contact the clinical director.

b If the potassium level rises, initially decrease/discontinue any potassium supplementation or downtitrate the aldosterone antagonist if one is being used. Recheck the potassium level in 1–2 days. If the potassium level remains elevated >5.0, try increasing/initiating a loop diuretic, recheck the level the next day, and contact the clinical director. Stop the ACE inhibitor if potassium is >5.5 and recheck the next day.

6 After achieving the target dose or the maximum tolerated ACE inhibitor dose, the patient can be monitored at regular clinic visits.

7 If the patient does not tolerate agent used because of rash or cough, stop the ACE inhibitor and contact the medical director. An ACE inhibitor rechallenge can be contemplated with the same or another ACE inhibitor. Consider using ARBs or hydralazine and nitrates for ACE inhibitor intolerant patients.

ARBs can be substitutes or supplements to ACE inhibitor therapy. Again, how and when to use ARBs is the purview of the medical director, who will lay out the therapeutic strategy for the patient at the index visit that initiates the "incident to" drug titration visits.

ARB protocol

1 Only two ARBs have proven efficacy in HF. Diovan (valsartan) has a target dose of 160 mg b.i.d. Atacand (candesartan) has a target dose of 32 mg q.d.

2 Obtain baseline renal function and serum electrolytes prior to initiating ACE inhibitor. Repeat renal function and chemistry analysis 1 week after an increase in dose, or if symptoms occur. A Bio-Z can also be obtained if there is a question as to whether the patient will tolerate the next dose titration.

3 Start titration at one-fourth to one-half of the target dose and titrate upward every other week as clinical symptoms, blood pressure, and laboratory results allow.

4 Monitor blood pressure and clinical symptoms during titration via clinic visits or telemanagement. Do not uptitrate unless BP is stable and is >90 mm Hg systolic.

5 Evaluate electrolyte and blood urea nitrogen/creatinine levels during the titration phase:

    a If the creatinine level rises 0.5 mg/dL, contact the clinical director.

    b If the potassium level rises, initially decrease/discontinue any potassium supplementation or downtitrate the aldosterone antagonist if one is being used. Recheck the potassium level in 1–2 days. If the potassium level remains elevated >5.0, try increasing/initiating a loop diuretic, recheck the level the next day, and contact the clinical director. Stop the ARB if potassium is >5.5 and recheck the next day.

6 After achieving the target dose or the maximum tolerated dose, the patient can be monitored at regular clinic visits.

The combination of hydralazine and nitrates was clearly established for black patients with HF in the AHeFT trial. Questions for the medical director are when to use this combination in nonblack patients and whether to use the therapy as a substitute for ACE inhibitors or ARBs in the presence of renal insufficiency or hyperkalemia. There is also the question whether to use BiDil, the proprietary formulation, or generic equivalents. The FDA has indicated that these two strategies are not equivalent. If you decide to use BiDil, then an appropriate protocol would be:

Hydralazine/nitrate protocol

1 BiDil is the combination of hydralazine and isosorbide dinitrate. Each tablet contains 37.5 mg of hydralazine and 20 mg isosorbide dinitrate. The target dose is two pills t.i.d. (hydralazine 75 mg t.i.d. and isosorbide dinitrate 40 mg t.i.d.).

2 No bloodwork needs to be monitored during BiDil titration. Only symptoms (fatigue, dizziness, and headache) and hemodynamics need to be monitored. Blood pressure monitoring might be sufficient, but Bio-Z measurements can be used if the ability of the patient to tolerate the next dose is a concern.

3 The starting dose of BiDil is one pill t.i.d. In fragile patients a half pill t.i.d. can be used.

4 The dose can be increased as rapidly as every 3–5 days. Increasing the dose every 2 weeks is more typical. Uptitration should wait until side effects resolve.

5 Because of the nitrate component of BiDil, some drugs for erectile dysfunction cannot be used.

6 If generic hydralazine/nitrate therapy is to be used, start both the nitrates and the hydralazine simultaneously. It may also be important to take the two medications at the same time of day. The use of nitrate patches or isosorbide mononitrate with hydralazine has not been studied in HF.

Dose titration of generic hydralazine

Starting dose	Steps	Target dose
25 mg b.i.d.	25 mg t.i.d., 50 mg t.i.d.	75 mg t.i.d.

Dose titration of isosorbide dinitrate

Starting dose	Steps	Target dose
20 mg t.i.d.	As allowed by symptoms	40 mg t.i.d.

Aldosterone antagonists are part of the neurohormonal blockade that is the basis of HF therapy today. In the absence of close monitoring, you can expect that some of your HF patients will get into trouble with aldosterone antagonists. Even with monitoring, there will be some cases of serious hyperkalemia, but hopefully your monitoring will head off some of these problems.

Aldosterone antagonists protocol

1 Spironolactone has been shown to prolong life in HF patients. The target dose is 25 mg q.d., although higher doses can be used if a patient has a problem with hypokalemia. Inspira (eplerenone) is a second-generation aldosterone antagonist, with a target dose of 50 mg q.d. It has been tested in post-myocardial infarction left ventricular dysfunction, but not in HF per se. It has none of the estrogen-like side effects of spironolactone, so it is used if spironolactone produces gynecomastia or erectile dysfunction.

2 The starting dose of spironolactone is 12.5 mg q.d. or 25 mg q.o.d. Inspira is started at 25 mg q.d., with a single-step titration to the target dose of 50 mg q.d. The focus during titration is on side effects and monitoring potassium. Consider tapering down oral potassium supplementation with initiation of spironolactone and/or during use. Potassium levels should be monitored:

  a Day 1: Serum potassium should be measured before initiating therapy

  b Week 1: Measure 1 week after start of treatment dose or dose adjustment

  c Month 1: Measure again 1 month after start of treatment or dose adjustment

  d Every 3 months thereafter

  Patients at particular risk are those with baseline renal insufficiency and those with diabetic nephropathy.

3 Dose adjustments are based on potassium levels. For eplerenone, the adjustment protocol is:

Serum potassium (mEq/L)	Action	Dose adjustment
< 5.0	Increase	25 mg q.o.d. to 25 mg q.d. 25 mg q.d. to 50 mg q.d.
5.0–5.4	Maintain	No adjustment
5.5–5.9	Decrease	50 mg q.d. to 25 mg q.d. 25 mg q.d. to 25 mg q.o.d. 25 mg q.o.d. to withhold
≥6.0	Withhold and notify clinical director	

4 If creatinine level rises 0.5 mg/dL during the titration process, consider tapering down the dosage and/or frequency of spironolactone or discontinuing the spironolactone altogether. These agents do not cause renal function to deteriorate, but the efficacy of spironolactone if serum creatinine is >2.5 mg/dL is unknown.

The medical therapy that seems to have made the most impact on HF patient outcomes in my opinion is the emergence of β-blocker therapy. When I was in training, the use of β-blockers in HF was malpractice. Now they have the highest level of recommendation in both sets of national guidelines. Initially there was fear of using these agents in the setting of HF, so initiation was done with great trepidation, doses were raised slowly, and monitoring was done in prolonged office visits. Today things are a little more relaxed. However, most referrals I receive find patients on low doses of non-evidence-based β-blockers. Needless to say, this is one of the most important drug protocols for an HF program.

β-Blockers protocol

1 Carvedilol at a dose ≥6.25 mg b.i.d. can be considered for all HF patients. Toprol XL 200 mg q.d. and bisoprolol 10 mg q.d. can be considered for patients with moderate HF.
2 β-blockers should not be initiated in patients who:
  a Are in a fluid overloaded state
  b Are hypotensive (<80 mm Hg systolic)
  c Are in acute decompensated HF
  d Have heart block or other conduction abnormalities
3 Prior to initiation of β-blockers:
  a Review current medications for use of other β-blockers (e.g., eye drops).
  b Review patient's medical history for a history of or risk for β-blocker intolerance (COPD, asthma, diabetes, bradycardia, hypotension, etc.).
  c Record NYHA classification, LVEF (left ventricular ejection fraction), and vital signs.
  d Obtain a recent history for worsening HF (edema, weight gain, etc.) to make sure patient is stable before β-blocker initiation.
  e Educate the patient that signs and symptoms of HF (dyspnea, edema, etc.) may become worse during the titration process and usually will subside within 8–10 weeks, but if such symptoms occur, they should call the HF clinic staff.

4 Educate the patient on the possible effects of β-blockers on diabetic control, hyperlipidemia, and pulmonary status, and their need to report changes to the HF team.

Carvedilol titration

1 Initiate Coreg (carvedilol) at 3.125 mg b.i.d. and double the dose every 2 weeks to 6.25 mg b.i.d., 12.5 mg b.i.d., and then to 25 mg b.i.d. for optimal dosing. The target dose is at least 6.25 mg b.i.d. Uptitrate if the patient has had no exacerbation of symptoms, HR (heart rate) is >50 bpm, and systolic BP is >85 mm Hg.

2 Goal dosing in HF patients:

  a Carvedilol 25 mg b.i.d. for patients weighing <187 lb

  b Carvedilol 50 mg b.i.d. for patients weighing >187 lb

3 Titration process may be lengthened according to individual patient responses (fatigue, dyspnea, edema, hypotension, and bradycardia). Consider increasing only the evening dose, utilizing a "half-step titration" for patients who are poorly tolerating the titration protocol.

4 For patients not tolerating the β-blocker titration:

  a Separate the timing of the ACE inhibitor dose and β-blocker by at least 2 hours during the day. Consider a once daily ACE inhibitor, which can be taken q.h.s.

  b Downtitrate the ACE inhibitor or other hypotensive agent.

  c Follow weights closely and up- or downtitrate diuretics accordingly.

  d Administer carvedilol with food to slow absorption.

5 Instruct the patient not to take the β-blocker immediately prior to a clinic visit so that a dosage adjustment decision may be made and observed in the clinic that day.

  a If the patient does take the β-blocker within 2 hours of a titration visit, administer only half the new dose for that visit (so that the clinic visit dose and the dose already taken by the patient add up to the new dose).

  b If the patient takes a β-blocker dose within 2–5 hours of a titration visit, consider rescheduling the visit if the patient has been particularly fragile.

Toprol XL titration

1 For Toprol XL (metoprolol succinate), begin at 25 mg q.d. (12.5 mg in more severe HF patients), then double the dose every 2 weeks until achieving the target dose of 200 mg/day, or the maximum dose tolerated.

2 The minimally effective dose is unknown, but is >100 mg. If intolerable symptoms (e.g., exacerbation of bronchospastic lung disease, loss of glycemic control in a brittle diabetic) at subtarget doses of Toprol XL, consider switching to carvedilol with a target dose ≥6.25 mg b.i.d.

Bisoprolol titration

1 Bisoprolol should be initiated at 1.25 mg q.d.

2 Uptitrations can occur every 2 weeks. The target dose is 10 mg q.d.; 5 mg q.d. may not confer a benefit to HF patients.

3 If intolerable symptoms (e.g., exacerbation of bronchospastic lung disease, loss of glycemic control in a brittle diabetic) at subtarget doses of bisoprolol, consider switching to carvedilol with a target dose >6.25 mg b.i.d.

It is difficult to anticipate all the needs that individual patients will present to your staff during clinic visits and telemanagement contacts. New staff, in particular, can be hesitant to titrate drug therapy in patients as sick as the patients in your clinic will be. An additional aid my staff has found helpful is a symptom assessment tool. This can be quickly gathered on each patient contact and used to decide whether to proceed with drug titration. A symptom score <30 usually means that it is safe to proceed with drug uptitration. If the score exceeds 30, the medical director or clinical director probably needs to be consulted. We also tell the staff that even if the symptom score is ≤30, but systolic BP is <95 mm Hg or HR is <60 bpm, they should still notify medical director or clinical director.

HF Symptom Assessment

Scoring scale: (good health = 1) 1, 2, 3, 4, 5 (poor health = 5)

1 How would rate your overall health?
   1, 2, 3, 4, 5
2 How did you sleep last night?
   1, 2, 3, 4, 5
3 How is your breathing?
   1, 2, 3, 4, 5
4 How is your swelling?
   1, 2, 3, 4, 5
5 How is your appetite?
   1, 2, 3, 4, 5
6 How many pounds is your weight above target?
   −3, −2, −1, 0, 1, 2, 3, 4, 5, . . .
7 How is your energy level?
   1, 2, 3, 4, 5

8 Have you had dizziness or passed out?
 1, 2, 3, 4, 5
Score:
 <10 Great!
 10 to 25 OK
 26 to 30 Intensified follow-up will be needed
 • **31 Action required; contact the medical or clinical director**

Additional Questions:
Have you been hospitalized since our last contact?
What is your weight?
What is your BP?
What is your heart rate?
What was your fluid intake yesterday?
What was your sodium intake yesterday?
What medicines do you take?

One of the shifts in therapy over the last few years has been the role of digoxin. While once a pillar of HF therapy, the DIG trial showed that digoxin does not convey a survival benefit. A DIG trial substudy even showed that in women digoxin may worsen survival. It was also revealed that digoxin levels should be kept <1.0 because of safety concerns. Digoxin is still used, but is best applied to men with advanced symptomatic disease.

Digoxin protocol

1 Digoxin is used for symptom relief in men with advanced HF:
 a Cardiothoracic ratio >0.5 on CXR
 b LVEF <25%
 c NYHA Class III/IV
2 The starting dose and target dose is 0.125 mg q.d. Some patients, especially elderly patients, may need the dose reduced to 0.125 mg q.o.d.
3 The digoxin level should be ≤1.0.
4 Digoxin needs to be monitored carefully in the presence of renal insufficiency.
5 Hold the digoxin if significant hyperkalemia or hypokalemia develops until the problem is resolved.

> **6** The long-term use of digoxin increases the incidence of estrogen-like side effects from spironolactone.

Another therapy for symptom relief is diuretic therapy. In the early days of HF disease management, it was felt that a major value of the program was to proactively search out early signs of volume overload, and then use intensified diuretic therapy to avert a future HF hospitalization. While an HF program now has many other functions, helping patients self-manage their diuretic therapy is still an important activity. Until patients reach independence in this area, your staff will need a protocol for diuretic therapy as well.

Diuretic therapy protocol

Drugs	Doses
Furosemide	20 mg q.d. to 320 mg b.i.d.
Bumetanide	1 mg q.d. to 4 mg b.i.d.
Torsemide	10 mg q.d. to 200 mg q.d.
Metolazone	2.5 mg q.d. to 10.0 mg q.d.

1 Diuretics provide symptom relief. They generally do not prolong life.

2 Furosemide has poor bioavailability. It works best if taken in the fasting state and if the patient can remain supine for at least 1 hour after taking it. Bumetanide and torsemide have better bioavailability.

3 Diuretics are threshold drugs. Once a dose is found that induces diuresis, more frequent dosing (rather than higher single doses) is usually required to mobilize more fluid.

4 If metolazone is used, it may be more effective if given 30 minutes before a loop diuretic.

5 Before starting a diuretic, check a basic metabolic profile (BMP). Make sure that the K^+ is over 3.5 before intensifying diuretic therapy.

> For K^+ < 4.0, give 20 mEq KCl/day
> For K^+ < 3.5, give 40 mEq KCl/day and recheck BMP in 1 day
> For K^+ < 3.0, give 80 mEq KCl/day and recheck BMP in 1 day

6 Repeat the BMP after 2 days if the diuretics is increased to see if K^+ supplementation is needed. Hold the diuretic if the K^+ is ≤ 3.0.

For K^+ < 4.0, give 20 mEq KCl/day
For K^+ < 3.5, give 40 mEq KCl/day and recheck BMP in 2 days
For K^+ < 3.0, give 80 mEq KCl/day and recheck BMP in 1 day

7 When metolazone is added to a loop diuretic, K^+ supplementation should be doubled and a BMP checked after 3 days of combination therapy.

For K^+ < 4.0, give an extra 20 mEq KCl/day
For K^+ < 3.5, give an extra 40 mEq KCl/day and recheck BMP in 2 days
For K^+ < 3.0, give an extra 80 mEq KCl/day and recheck BMP in 1 day

8 Aldosterone antagonists can be used instead of K^+ supplementation.
9 The short-term goal with diuretic therapy is to relieve symptoms and return to dry weight. The long-term goal is to make diuretics p.r.n. if possible and, in any case, to have the patient self-manage his or her diuretics.
10 Dose adjustment is based on daily weights, edema, and dyspnea. If the weight rises 3 lb above target in 1 day, or 5 lb above target over a week, the patient should take an extra dose of loop diuretic. If the weight is >5 lb above target, 2.5–5.0 mg metolazone q.d. 30 minutes before the loop diuretic can be added.
11 Metolazone should be taken until the weight is <5 lb above target.
12 If hypokalemia is refractory, check a serum magnesium level. If Mg^{2+} is less than normal, give $MgSO_4$, 3 g IVPB or MgO, 3 g p.o. Follow this with Slow Mag, one tablet q.d. or b.i.d. Repeat Mg^{2+} level in 1 week.

HF is a chronic disease. Unlike pneumonia, where a patient becomes ill, is treated, and then the condition resolves, HF is characterized by an ongoing series of exacerbations and stabilizations. Drug therapy is therefore an ongoing effort, with doses being intensified at one point and dialed back at another. Once your staff becomes experienced at matching the intensity of the disease process with the intensity of therapy, you will be far ahead in managing your patients and reducing unnecessary hospitalizations.

Summary

Initiating, up- and downtitrating the life-prolonging HF drug therapies is a major activity of the HF clinic. For the reasons discussed earlier, the bulk of the optimization of the medical regimen is done by nonphysicians. Your program will use drug treatment protocols to implement the therapies chosen for a patient by the medical director. These protocols do not select the therapies a patient should be on, the order of the therapies to be applied, or which therapies should be used together. Again, this is the role of the medical director, and protocols do not replace that responsibility. Rather the protocols lay out how to meet the patient goals laid out by the medical director.

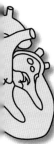

CHAPTER 13

Telemanagement algorithms

The current healthcare environment demands that superior care be delivered at a lower cost. The best way to leverage your personnel is the telemanagement of heart failure. Here we will discuss how to construct your own telemanagement protocols to detect problems, and treatment protocols that you can use for intervention.

In calculating financial projections in an earlier chapter, I discussed leveraging your resources as a way to assure the profitability of your HF disease management program. The emphasis then was to identify your growth-limiting resource (usually physician resources) and then working on leveraging that resource. As your program grows, the clinical director also becomes stretched, so strategies for leveraging his or her time will also need to be developed. Eventually you will need to leverage your HF nurses as well. One method of gaining such leverage for nursing resources is telemanagement. By using a telephone instead of a clinic visit for patient contact, the number of contacts can be inexpensively and substantially increased.

Telemanagement alone has been shown to decrease hospitalizations and increase patient compliance, but this is not a replacement for your HF clinic. Hospitals that I have seen attempt to run a virtual HF clinic via phone have found that this generally works only for the very ill patient, and even then management is difficult when there are no face-to-face contacts whatsoever to bind the patient and the caregiver in a therapeutic relationship. Telemanagement should supplement rather than replace the program–patient relationship and extend the educational process begun in your office.

Once an effective telemanagement program is up and running, it may decrease the need for other parts of your program. For example, earlier we discussed the role of group visits in a contemporary HF program. In addition to the CHCC (Community Health Continuity Clinic) model that provides continuing care, I described the DIGMA (drop-in group medical appointment) model to deal with episodic care, providing patients ready access to care at the early stages of a clinical problem. The DIGMA groups are very helpful early in an HF program's life. With frequent and professional telemanagement, though, I have found that problems are so well taken care of that the DIGMA groups become less utilized, and sometimes can be eliminated.

Again, telephone contact leverages not only physician resources, but also staff resources. Depending upon the information to be obtained, the staff making the patient contact could be a medical assistant (MA), nurse, or practitioner with an advanced degree. If the call is to record daily weight and administer a symptom questionnaire, then the MA would be appropriate. A weight gain of 2 lb in a day or 5 lb in a week would trigger a call from a nurse, so that protocol-driven adjustment of medical therapy could be undertaken. A complex or fragile patient might need to have contact with a nurse practitioner or physician assistant.

Over the last decade, large-scale telemanagement systems have been developed that allow the physician to outsource these services. These systems utilize a centralized panel of nurses to provide telemanagement services for patients dispersed across the country. Another option is the digital self-reporting telemanagement system that allows patients to enter daily reports about their current state of health which are then analyzed by an HF team or by intelligent databases to identify early signs of patient decompensation.

Telephone management guidelines

1 Patients will receive a telephone encounter within 48 h of hospital discharge or referral to the HF program.

2 Patients at risk for noncompliance or rehospitalization will receive a telephone encounter at least once a week. If weight or symptoms of HF are increasing or the patient shows misunderstanding of or noncompliance with the medical regimen, an HF nurse should also call the patient.

3 An encounter with a home healthcare agency nurse visiting the patient may be utilized as a patient telephone encounter equivalent.

4 For stable, lower risk patients, the frequency of telephone encounters can be decreased to monthly or bimonthly.

A patient is considered stable when:

a Target weight has been maintained for 2 wk

b No complaints of increased dyspnea or edema

c Decreasing or unchanging peripheral edema

d Medications have been stable for the last 2 wk

e Patient or family is able to list the signs and symptoms of increasing HF, as well as the medication list and the role of each medicine (e.g., when to take metolazone or to increase the loop diuretic)

5 Patient and family will be instructed to initiate a telephone encounter when they note the occurrence of any of the signs and symptoms of HF listed on the "When to call us" list.

The telemanagement encounter

What you include in a telephone contact is determined by the scope and treatment style of your program. You will want to know if any benchmark events have occurred; e.g., has the patient been hospitalized since the last contact or have there been any changes in medications. The three most important measurements you need on a day-to-day basis are the patient's weight, blood pressure (if you can get it), and the level of HF signs and symptoms. You then use these three variables to determine if a patient is stable or if intervention (via telephone or in the HF clinic) is necessary.

In the last chapter, I presented a tool to assess HF symptoms. Your program may want to follow different parameters. For illustration purposes, let's construct a telemanagement encounter protocol for XYZ HF program.

Principles of telemanagement contacts: initial level contacts

- Decide upon a small number of parameters to measure.
- Use the KISS principle so that data collection can be done by:
  —Patients themselves
  —Nonphysicians
  —Case managers with a large caseload
- Responses should be weighted to allow development of triggers that initiate an intervention.

To keep things simple, you may still want to use the approach of the HF symptom assessment tool from the last chapter and assign point scores to patient responses during a telemanagement encounter. The total score can be used by the staff members to determine if the patient is getting into trouble and when other staff need to be consulted (e.g., when the MA needs to contact the nurse, when the nurse needs to contact the clinical director).

For a patient's body weight, your staff member will need to collect and compare today's weight, previous weights, and the patient's target weight. Points can be assigned to the change in body weight:

- 0 points if at target weight
- 1 point if ≤ 2 lb over target weight
- 2 points if >2 lb over target weight
- 4 points if 5 lb over target weight or if >3 lb weight gain in 1 day

Note that the point scale need not be linear; e.g., there is no body weight that results in a score of 3 points. Symptoms can also be weighted. For dyspnea, a scoring system could be:

- 0 points if no dyspnea
- 1 point if dyspneic while:

—walking one flight of stairs
—walking 100 ft
—taking out the garbage
—gardening
—carrying groceries
• 3 points if dyspneic while:
—making a bed
—getting dressed
—shampooing hair
—brushing teeth
—putting on shoes
• 4 points if dyspneic at rest or for a change in dyspnea compared to yesterday

By its very nature, telemanagement focuses on HF symptoms, but HF signs can also be scored. However, to be usable in a telemanagement setting, the signs need to be measured in a way that lends itself to self-assessment by the patient. Edema is one such physical sign which can be scored this way:
• 0 points for no edema
• 1 point for pitting edema
• 2 points for loss of ankle anatomy or tight fit on clothes, shoes, rings
• 4 points for edema to the knee or a change from yesterday

In the telemanagement contact, one would want to keep the parameters (signs, symptoms, weight) to less than 12. The scores from the 12 questions you devise are then used to decide if an interventional contact should be made. Triggers to contact a patient may be:
• Any question scoring 4 points
• A total score over 25 points
• Any patient not reached by phone
• Any patient who feels an ED (emergency department) visit is on the horizon
• If a patient is confused or upset about medications, his or her HF status or progress, or his or her relationship with your HF program.

Once a patient is assessed, a decision needs to be made about the need for intervention. These interventions need to be standardized. An example of telemanagement protocols is given below:

Telephonic patient encounter algorithm

1 With each patient encounter, an encounter form will be completed and will become part of the patient's record.

---

2 Patient's current and target weight should be compared.

3 A symptom history will be obtained. Dyspnea, orthopnea, paroxysmal nocturnal dyspnea, activity tolerance/fatigue, and edema will be recorded on the encounter form.

4 A medication history will note any changes in the medical regimen and missed doses.

Intervening for changes in patient status

Mild changes

5 If it is determined that the patient has experienced *mild* deterioration of HF, the therapeutic interventions will be:

a Reinforce medical/dietary compliance; review the medication list with the patient.

b Instruct patient/family as to when to call/page the HF team with any further changes.

c Instruct patient/family on emergency interventions (EMS-911).

d Follow-up telemanagement daily for 3 days. An HF nurse will be notified to consider an HF clinic visit or change in medication.

Moderate changes

6 If it is determined that the patient has experienced *moderate* deterioration of HF, the HF nurse will make contact. The therapeutic interventions will be:

a Take 2.5–5.0 mg of metolazone, followed 30 min later by a dose of a loop diuretic.

b If the patient has no metolazone, the patient is to take an extra dose of diuretic for 2 days.

c Potassium replacement: In patients without evidence of renal compromise (increased creatinine, renal failure, increased serum K^+ levels, etc.) instruct patient to take an extra 20–40 mEq of KCl now and an extra 20–40 mEq the next day.

d Reinforce medical/dietary compliance. Review medications and optimize angiotensin-converting enzyme (ACE) inhibitor if BP is known.

e Instruct patient/family to call/page the HF team with any further changes.

f Instruct patient/family on emergency interventions (EMS-911).

g Instruct patient to come to the HF clinic within 1–2 days for adjustment of the medical regimen.

h Telephone management daily until patient is seen in clinic.

Severe changes

7 If it is determined that the patient has experienced a *significant* deterioration of HF, an HF nurse will contact the patient and consider the following interventions:

  a Metolazone 5.0–10.0 mg now, followed by a dose of a loop diuretic in 30 min. If metolazone is not available then instruct patient to take an extra dose of loop diuretic.

  b Potassium replacement: In patients without evidence of renal compromise (increased creatinine, renal failure, increased serum K^+ levels, etc.) instruct patient to take an extra 20–40 mEq of KCl now and an extra 20–40 mEq the next day.

  c Clinic visit as soon as possible (same day).

  d i.v. diuretic and/or inotrope infusion in the infusion suite.

  e Optimize ACE inhibitor (increase dose one-step toward target dose) if BP is >90 mm Hg systolic.

  f EMS-911 or closest ER (emergency room) immediately if symptoms meet previously described criteria.

  g Notify clinical or medical director.

  h Recheck the patient via telephone in 1 h.

Outsourcing telemanagement

You may feel your staff is too small or too busy to provide consistent telemanagement services to your patients. Outsourcing telemanagement is one alternative to providing this service yourself. There are many disease management companies that utilize nurses to staff a central phone bank that reaches out to HF patients throughout the country to deliver protocol-driven care. When a patient needs to be seen, a home health nurse is sent to the patient's home. Because the physician is not a part of the care, I have sometimes had difficulty coordinating my treatment plan and style with the telemanagement provided by such companies. Presenting a consistent treatment plan to the patient from my program and the telemanagement nurse from another organization can be very challenging at times.

Other HF disease management companies take a different approach. These companies rely on patient self-monitoring and collect patient self-reports into a database on a computer in your office or in the company offices. The database is reviewed daily by your nurses or the company's nurses and therapy is adjusted by protocol. Typically, these protocols can be customized by you to reflect your priorities and treatment styles. The self-monitoring device varies from company to company. One company places a device in the patient's home which uses voice prompts that direct the patient to weigh himself or herself on the scale that is part of the device, to obtain a blood pressure, heart rate, and oxygen saturation, again using accessories connected to the patient monitor. A quality-of-life questionnaire is also administered by voice prompts. These data are transmitted wirelessly to the computer installed in your office. A similar system utilizes a standing scale that transmits data via a modem from the back of the scale. A unique feature of this system is that the handles of the scale measure bioimpedance to get a measure of thoracic fluid content. The monitoring provided by these systems is quite sophisticated.

These services are expensive, costing up to hundreds of dollars per patient per month, but can be effective. If targeted to your sickest patients, they can be a cost-effective alternative. However, because of reimbursement issues, systems such as these typically target hospitals and payors as their customers rather than private practices.

Managing medications by phone

I've presented some of the protocols that I've seen used for patient management, as well as a framework for developing telemanagement protocols. Your own protocols have to reflect your program's treatment style and the interests and abilities of your staff. We use symptom scores, body weight, and BP to decide how a patient is doing over the telephone. Your HF staff will need to be trained as to how you want clinical decisions to be made.

Some HF programs use more aggressive protocols, initiating and titrating ACE inhibitors and β-blockers at home as well as following patients' reported daily weights and blood pressures. Disease management programs far removed from patients, e.g., telephone banks of nurses in California managing patients across the country, may feel forced into such protocols to achieve desired clinical outcomes. That experience has made the medical community as a whole more comfortable expanding the use of telemanagement. I still think that it is important to touch the new HF patients frequently during the initial phases of the patients' experience to gain their confidence and to emphasize the pathway to their self-management. We touch more frequently with telemanagement these days, especially patients who travel long distances to see us or who are too sick to travel to the HF clinic. Nonetheless, I have found that we need to treat HF patients one at a time, and face-to-face encounters are an important part of that care. Telemanagement supplements but does not replace the face-to-face events. We have a low threshold for having a patient who is struggling at home to come in that day to the HF clinic.

Because of the close contact we maintain with our patients, there is usually no need to titrate ACE inhibitors or β-blockers in response to signs and symptoms revealed by telemanagement. In a very short time after program entry, most of our patients have had their chronic medical regimens optimized. We use telemanagement to continually tweak therapy to meet the day-to-day fluctuations of the patient's disease.

How intense should monitoring by telemanagement be?

When we first started following patients by phone, we started with a protocol based upon NYHA class. We called Class I patients once a quarter, Class II patients once a month, Class IIIA patients once a week, Class IIIB patients twice a week, and Class IV patients every other day (if they were not in our infusion suite or a hospice program). This inflexible approach did not work well for us. Our patients needed a more individualized approach irrespective of NYHA class. Some patients need more careful monitoring than others to keep out of trouble. While most patients are contacted at least once a month, I let the case managers set the intensity of monitoring beyond that.

Summary

Day-to-day management of HF in an aggressive, proactive manner is the strength of the disease management program approach. Using telemanagement and protocol-driven therapy, the patient's medical regimen is continually titrated. The parameters you use for these titrations, i.e., your telemanagement and drug therapy protocols, should reflect the philosophy and style of your program's approach to HF. Your protocols may well evolve over time as the training and experience of your staff increases, so that they can assume more autonomy in applying telemanagement protocols.

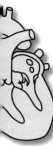

CHAPTER 14

Advanced therapies

We are continually developing new and better ways to treat HF. Every set of HF guidelines evaluates therapies that have emerged since the last set of guidelines were promulgated and casts an eye to new horizons that promise to bear fruit in the future. There comes a time when standard conventional therapies are not enough, especially in patients with advanced HF. If yours is to be a full-service HF program, then you will want to consider which of these promising approaches you should incorporate.

In any chronic, lethal incurable disease that is as common as HF there will be ongoing significant research into new ways to battle the disease. This will include both pharmacologic as well as nonpharmacologic therapies. In this chapter we will consider some of these advanced therapies.

The infusion suite

The infusion suite is where you administer the most potent therapies to the sickest of your patients. Issues of informed consent, advance directives, and protocols for the initiation and continuation of such therapies are critical issues your program will need to address. At one point, the main activity of the outpatient infusion suite was to administer inotropic therapy to NYHA Class IIIB/IV patients to provide enough symptom relief to avoid a hospitalization. Intravenous inotropes do not prolong life. They only reduce symptoms. They may even shorten survival. Patients will need to have a clear understanding of this before undergoing such therapy. This goes beyond written consent; patients must give truly informed consent.

With the advent of β-blockers, nitrate-enhancing therapies, etc., the need for inotropes has diminished. This therapy always applied only to a minority of patients in an HF program. Now it is a smaller minority. There is general agreement that acute inotropic support in the CCU (coronary care unit) is helpful in the right patient cohort. There is also general agreement that daily use of high-dose inotropes, whether i.v. or p.o., shortens survival. There is intense disagreement as to where the risk/benefit lines cross. Discussions of the topic ignite intense emotions that are difficult to understand. Chronic, scheduled inotrope infusions are not recommended by the guidelines. The question remains open for short-term inotropes for decompensated patients.

Each program will need to decide for itself whether to offer inotropic therapy. In my program we did offer it to ill patients who had run out of options and were decompensated. Because we were quite upfront during our consent process that inotropes could adversely affect survival and because of the inconvenience of intravenous therapy, some patients declined this option. Others received either dobutamine or milrinone until their symptoms abated or they felt they had reached maximal benefit. We found that milrinone but not dobutamine had an impact on hospitalizations. Hospitalization rates in the year after inotrope support with milrinone was offered were one-third that of the previous year. Dobutamine provided no benefit, with hospitalization rates similar to that of patients who refused inotropic support.

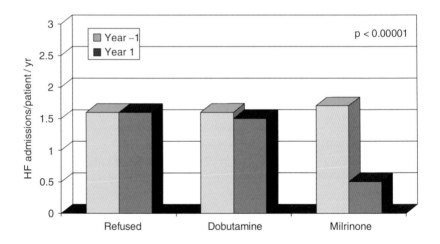

I am comfortable with short courses of milrinone—sparingly delivered—because of this experience. Inotropes are not the only infusion therapy of interest to HF patients. Nesiritide also had become adopted by many programs. Unlike the inotrope experience, though, with nesiritide we have some promising data in the high-risk patient subset of the FUSION trial. The subsequent FUSION-2 trial showed that the routine use of nesiritide for recently hospitalized HF patients did not reduce re-hospitalization rates. Like inotropes, then, infusions of nesiritide are not valuable as a preventive therapy, but instead are for the HF patient that has already decompensated. A meta-analysis of the nesiritide data suggested that the safety and efficacy of the therapy was not yet proven even for inpatients, so more work needed to be done. My personal experience has been that for some patients, nesiritide provided substantial benefit. Other patients, though, had little response. The next step for the medical community is to define the appropriate patient type for this therapy. As with inotropes, the emotional tone of discussions concerning outpatient nesiritide is unreasonable, unscientific, and confusing. Fortunately, unlike the story with inotropes, we will soon have a scientific answer for nesiritide.

The infusion suite can also be used for infusions of diuretic therapy. This has traditionally included only those few volume-overloaded patients who were resistant to oral loop diuretics and were responsive to continuous infusions of loop diuretics. A more intriguing use of the infusion suite for diuretic therapy may be the vasopressin antagonists that achieve aquaresis without upsetting K^+, etc. Outpatient studies have not yet been published, but this is another emerging therapy to watch.

Aquapheresis (ultrafiltration) is another effective therapy that also removes water without affecting electrolytes. Again, for a minority of patients, this is an attractive option. Although it is an invasive therapy, those experienced in the technique cite the only significant barrier to widespread adoption is the cost of the system and supplies.

External counterpulsation

A course of 35 one-hour outpatient external counterpulsation (ECP) treatments is currently indicated for the relief of refractory angina. A proposed mechanism of action is the stimulation of collateral formation. It would not seem a priori that ECP would have a role in the treatment of HF. In fact, the inflation of cuffs on the legs should induce venous return and could overwhelm the failing heart. It was surprising that in a registry of patients undergoing a course of ECP, some of the greatest benefit was seen in patients with left ventricular (LV) dysfunction. The enhanced ECP in HF pilot study was also encouraging. Unfortunately, results were mixed in the more definitive PEECH trial. I remain optimistic about ECP. I am most familiar with a single-center experience that prospectively measured NYHA class, a health satisfaction score (HSS), a 6-minute-walk (6MW) distance, left ventricular ejection fraction (LVEF), B-natriuretic peptide (BNP) levels, and the number of anginal episodes a week before and after a course of 34.6 ± 0.5 h of ECP in 53 adults with ischemic cardiomyopathy. ECP appeared to be beneficial:

	NYHA class	HSS	6MW	LVEF	BNP	Angina episodes per week
Baseline	2.7 ± 0.1	0.42 ± 0.02	907 ± 62	32 ± 1	306 ± 25	10 ± 2
Post-ECP	1.9 ± 0.1	0.62 ± 0.02	1090 ± 64	38 ± 2	263 ± 25	4 ± 1
p value	< 0.00001	< 0.00001	< 0.00001	< 0.00001	0.006	< 0.00001

This was not a randomized, placebo-controlled trial, but was prospective, using each patient as his or her own control. It seems to signal a clinical benefit in HF.

Device therapy

As an HF program, many of your patients will benefit from device therapy: either implantable cardioverter defibrillators or cardiac resynchronization therapy (CRT). Both these devices improve survival in HF. CRT also improves quality of life. The guidelines are fairly specific as to who you should refer for device therapy. I will assume that your electrophysiologist will do the implanting as well as the care and feeding of the devices from an electrical point of view. There are features of CRT monitoring that are of interest to the HF physician. As we discussed in a previous chapter, some Medtronic devices contain the OptiVol system to monitor patient volume status. In the figure below, the patient exhibits decreasing thoracic impedance in the upper panel, signifying better conduction in the chest, presumably from increased chest fluid. In lower panel, this is reflected in the OptiVol measurement. Toward the right hand side of the lower panel, the OptiVol measurement has crossed the threshold set by the physician. The upward trend in the OptiVol measurement suggests volume overload.

Some Guidant systems are enabled to be part of the Latitude home monitoring HF system. As this collects some of the same information you would collect normally through telemanagement, the Latitude system leverages your HF staff time. You will want to be sure that your program is able to access this data.

An emerging issue is the optimization of CRT systems. At the time of implantation, this is often done using a mathematical formula based on individual patient data. Over time, though, CRT should induce reverse remodeling of the failing heart. It has been suggested that the CRT system requires reoptimization every 3 months for the first few years after implant. Most often, CRT optimization is done using echocardiographic

The Medtronic OptiVol system

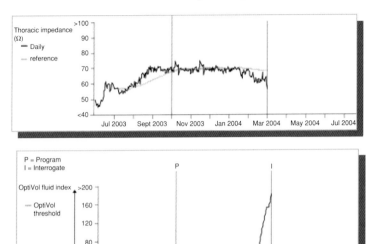

measurements such as the velocity time integral or, more recently, using echocardiographic assessment of LV dyssynchrony. While echocardiography is a reimbursable activity, in the current environment of downward pressure on revenues, it seems unlikely that a strategy of obtaining an echo every 3 months on CRT patients will be viewed favorably by payors. These echos are also time consuming.

In an earlier chapter, I proposed that at least two low-cost alternatives exist. The first is the Cardiodynamics Bio-Z system for noninvasive measurement of hemodynamics (in this case the preejection period and the left ventricular ejection time). The other is the Inovise Audicor TS (phonocardiogram) system (using the electromechanical activation time, EMAT, and the left ventricular systolic time, LVST). In my HF program, we compared these two low-cost approaches to echocardiography. The optimal atrioventricular (AV) delay suggested by the Bio-Z differed from echo by 38 ± 15 msec. The optimal AV delay suggested by the Audicor TS differed from echo by 25 ± 11 msec. These are well within our ability to program an AV delay. The simplicity of the Audicor TS in particular (but also the Bio-Z in experienced hands) is such that no physician time is required during testing. These systems are worth exploring further as our CRT population grows.

Audicor TS system

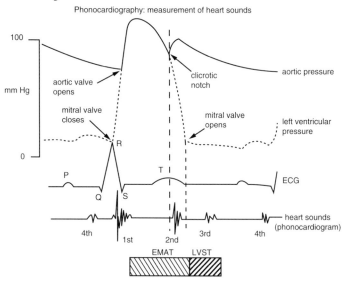

Phonocardiography: measurement of heart sounds

We have already discussed the Cardiodynamics Bio-Z system. The Inovise Audicor TS system takes a different approach to reach the same end, using electrocardiographic and phonocardiographic signals to assess LV performance. In the figure below, the EMAT and LVST measurements from the Audicor TS system taken at a variety of programmed AV delays agree

Optimizing CRT with the Audicor TS system

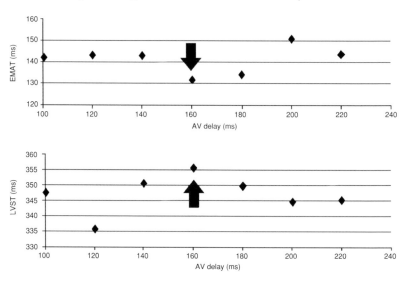

that 160 msec is the optimal AV delay of this particular CRT system at this point in time. Echocardiography suggested the same AV delay as optimal.

Summary

HF is a progressive illness, and so eventually many patients will cease to respond to traditional therapy. These are the patients who consume the most resources and are hospitalized the most often. The adoption of advanced therapies may be needed in your program to help those of these patients who are not candidates for transplantation. Some of these therapies are controversial, so you will need to evaluate how they apply to your patient population. They can also be costly, and yet result in a cost savings to the health care system.

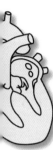

CHAPTER 15

Positioning your heart failure program as a center of expertise

All primary care physicians and cardiologists know how to take care of HF. Why should they use you or your HF program? Most general practices contain large cohorts of HF patients, and they are "doing just fine" taking care of these patients. The fact is, if they were doing just fine, HF would not be the leading reason for hospitalization of Medicare patients. How do you convince referral sources to utilize the program you've built? I have found referrals will come when you convince these physicians of four precepts.

There are many external forces influencing patient flow in the current healthcare environment. Traditional referral patterns, restricted payor panels, the location of your program, all have a bearing on your ultimate success. By focusing on four messages, I believe you will enjoy success once your doors are opened.

I. You enjoy taking care of heart failure patients. HF patients are a needy, resource consuming cohort, especially when the disease has advanced to NYHA Class III or IV. If you do not enjoy HF therapy, these patients are a burden to your practice, with frequent visits, frequent hospitalizations, frequent phone calls to the office, etc. By making it clear that these are the patients you want, you give an incentive for referrals to occur. These needy patients are the very patients who do best in a structured environment of education and monitoring. Not every patient will do well, but most improve dramatically in a disease management program based upon tele-management, education, and frequent office visits. Programs I have seen struggle are quick to see a patient and then turn the patient back over to the primary care physician with a list of suggestions, such as "begin a β-blocker and titrate to ___ mg." It is the hard work of slowly getting the patients on the right therapy that is so challenging. That is often what triggered the referral in the first place.

Once it's clear to your referral sources that you want this business, patients will find a way to you, even in today's health-care environment that restricts patients' access to services. The first referrals will be the sickest patients, but these are often the patients for which your program can do the most good. Later, as word of your enthusiasm for this subspecialty of cardiovascular medicine spreads, less sick patients will be referred. We commonly get referrals from cardiologists within and outside of our practice and have patients bypassing other programs to travel over 100 miles to come to us. Am I smarter than those other cardiologists? Hardly. It's our program and our enthusiasm for HF patient care that makes us attractive.

Equally important is making your program user-friendly. It must be painless for a referring physician to send you a patient. This means a friendly, "can do" receptionist and a staff that realizes that new patients must be seen quickly. It also means letters back to the referring doctors must be sent promptly and must reflect the enthusiasm and comprehensiveness of your care. Both the patient and referring physician need to come away with a pleasant experience, and know you are hungry for their business.

II. You are competent in heart failure care. You may enjoy HF therapy, but are you any good at it? The referring letters you send are opportunities to explain what care you are giving and why you are giving it. If, for example, you are changing captopril 25 mg t.i.d. to trandolapril 4 mg q.d., you can explain that trandolapril has the highest tissue penetration in vivo of any ACE inhibitor, increases compliance because of once-a-day dosing, has been shown in the longest clinical trial of ACE inhibitor therapy to benefit HF patients, and is a relatively low-cost therapy.

As the champion of your program, it is important to assume a public profile as an expert in HF in your medical community. This means speaking on HF to lay groups and to your peers. You need to speak enough that your program is automatically linked with HF in the community consciousness. This may mean "grand rounds" at your hospital not once a year, but twice a year. You may put on an HF symposium annually for your referring physicians. Much medical education now is done via industry-sponsored dinner programs or weekend events, and you will likely need to be on some of these speakers' bureaus.

When your hospital is redesigning its optimal pathway for HF admissions, you want to be on that committee. If the hospital is creating a program for inotrope infusions, you want to help in its design, even if you have an infusion suite. This may mean helping your competitors in providing HF care to their patients—it's true. The notion that you will garner 100% of the HF marketplace, though, is naive and unrealistic. It is important that you be a leader in all the HF initiatives. As a community leader in HF, you will be recognized as a competent caregiver in this area, and help define the community standard of care.

III. You do a better than average job. You enjoy HF medicine. You are competent in your care, but so are your referring physicians. You next need to show that your complicated and comprehensive HF program does a better than average job with HF therapy. This is hard to prove when you first open your doors. Soon, though, your periodic reassessments during benchmark visits can be compared to your baseline measurements, and you will have outcomes data to show.

The quickest data you can put together is data showing characteristics of your patients. For example, as already discussed, the first 100 patients in my first HF program were mostly NYHA Class III and IV. The average left ventricular ejection fraction (LVEF) was 22%. An early piece of analysis you can assemble can be a measure of your success in optimizing the medical regimen of your patients. Again, my results showed that our program intensified therapy:

Therapy	Baseline	1-yr follow-up
ACE inhibitors/ARBs	43	100
Digoxin	36	91
Diuretics	55	94
Triple therapy	21	90

By the end of our first year of operation, we could compare the number of hospital admissions in our cohort during the year prior to program entry with the number of hospitalizations in the year after entering our program. The 71% decrease in HF hospitalizations showed that we were doing something right—improving care in patients who were referred by other cardiologists.

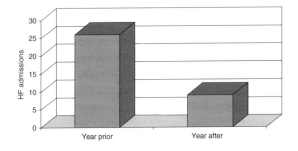

After a few years, we could show the benefit of our program to payors. One of our major hospitals experienced a steady decline in HF hospitalizations in the 2 years after initiating our program compared to the year before the program (Year −1).

Hospital one

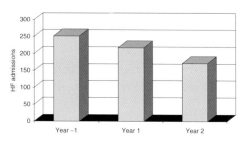

Interestingly, a similar-sized hospital 10 blocks away—where we had little presence—had the same patient mix, but HF hospitalizations at the second hospital did not change over the same time period, implying that our program was at least partly responsible for the difference seen at the first hospital.

Hospital two

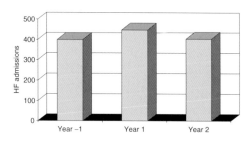

IV. You are state of the art. You are enthusiastic. You are competent. You even do a better than average job with HF patient care. Ultimately, you want to be the community resource on HF. You need to be state of the art, even if your program locally is not. To be an opinion leader for HF, you need to have an opinion on controversial areas of care.

For example, several small studies have shown that HF patients have a coenzyme Q10 (Co Q10) deficiency and that supplementation improves LVEF, 6-minute-walk-test results, and NYHA class. Other studies of Co Q10 show no benefit. Current guidelines do not recommend Co Q10 supplements in HF. As the local HF resource, you need to know this literature and have an opinion as to whether Co Q10 supplementation should be part of your protocols.

Another controversy revolves around the concomitant use of ACE inhibitor together with aspirin. A retrospective analysis of the VHeFT II,

CONSENSUS II, and SOLVD databases with enalapril, the HOPE and AIRE studies with ramipril, and the SAVE trial with captopril showed disturbing results. In fact, in the SOLVD study, if you were an HF patient on an antiplatelet agent like aspirin, you were worse off if you were on the ACE inhibitor than if you were on placebo. In the GUSTO I and EPILOG trials, mortality was higher in patients treated with ACE inhibitor and aspirin as compared to those treated with aspirin alone. The combination roughly doubled the risk of death. The data is retrospective and controversial, but you need to evaluate the literature and decide if aspirin is a good idea for your HF patients or if they would be better off, for example, on clopidogrel as a platelet inhibitor (which does not interact with ACE inhibitor). Another idea is to reduce the ASA dose in HF patients. However, in our program we started testing for aspirin resistance and found that over half of our HF patients did not respond to 81 mg ASA q.d. Current guidelines recommend against the use of NSAIDs because of this issue. The HFSA guidelines suggest not using ASA in nonischemic cardiomyopathy for the same reason. What you do in your community may depend on how you feel after you review the data.

An emerging body of data suggests sleep disturbances are common in HF patients and nocturnal oxygen or continuous positive airway pressure may be helpful in improving LVEF and NHYA class. Guidelines support screening for sleep apnea. How it should be handled is not clear. There is no definitive answer yet; you need to be an opinion leader guiding your referring physicians as to how to apply the available information. As I discussed in the opening chapters, you are the trail guide.

You may also find it helpful to be a pioneer, and involve your program in HF research. Clinical trials of vasopressin antagonists, endothelin antagonists, and vasopeptidase inhibitors have been frustrating, but ongoing trials will shape our future treatment algorithms. I have found participation in clinical research trials to be a significant source of professional satisfaction. This effort also represents an alternative source of revenue to help your program thrive. Most importantly, an active research program keeps your staff intellectually alert and curious, so that it is easier to continually reinvent your program through a process of continuous quality improvement. Your patients end up with the best of care.

Partnering

Your program may benefit from joint programs with your hospital, insurance payors, or industry. If there is a sleep lab in your community, your HF program may well become one of its major referral sources, so a partnership would logically follow. In addition to speaking engagements, your staff may participate in health fairs or employer programs. These partnerships can raise your program's visibility in the community and can also shift some of the costs of implementing and marketing your program, especially in its start-up phase.

There is certainly enough work to go around to justify partnering with others interested in HF care.

Best of luck with your program!

Index

About the Author

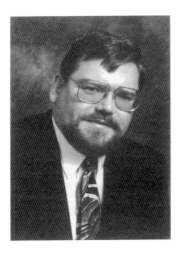

Michael McIvor, MD received his cardiology training at the Johns Hopkins Hospital and was a research fellow at the National Institutes of Health, studying cellular electrophysiology, electromechanical coupling in the myocyte, and autonomic modulation of cardiac function. He entered private medical practice as an interventional cardiologist in 1989 and proceeded to build disease management programs lipidology and heart failure as well as programs in clinical research and medical education. Dr McIvor has authored more than 50 publications in peer-reviewed journals, has written four books and is a nationally recognized speaker.

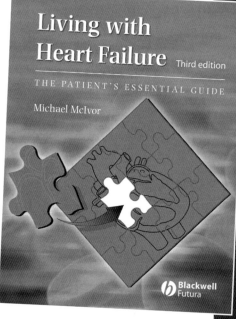